Alzheimer's

Are You At Risk?

A Roadmap and Guide to the
Cause, Prevention and Treatment
of Alzheimer's Disease

by
David A. Howe MD, DC

The information in this book is based on science yet written for the lay person in easy to understand language. Advice herein is intended for informational purposes only. Book is meant to help readers better understand dementia and Alzheimer's health concerns. Information is based on review of scientific research data, historical practice patterns, and clinical experience. This information should not be interpreted as specific medical advice. Users should consult with a qualified healthcare provider for specific questions regarding therapies, diagnosis and/or health conditions prior to making therapeutic decisions.

For general information on products and services, or for technical support, please contact NutraGen™ Customer Service Department within the United States at (877) 417-7873 or write to NutraGen™ Health Innovations, Inc., 10366 Roselle Street, Suite A, San Diego, CA 92121. For immediate information and product referral go to www.nutragen.com.

To contact Dr. Howe directly you can access his website www.stemcells4life.net, email info@stemcells4life.net. Subscribe here for the latest updates and news.

ISBN-13: 978-1543266924
ISBN-10: 1543266924

Printed in the United States of America
Available from Amazon.com, or directly from www.Stemcells4life.net and NutraGen™ Health Innovations, Inc., www.nutragen.com.

Back cover photo by Domminique Cognee, www.cogneephotography.com, Greenwood, California, Specializing in portraiture's and equine events.

Summer 2017

CONTENT

PART FOUR

Resolution – The Good News

PART FIVE

JumpStart

APPENDIX

Introduction

Some say you cannot have life both ways. You either die young or, if you live long enough, age related slow-down commonly known as dementia becomes a normal consequence.

In 1950 the US average age hovered around 65.4. Today men live to age 76+ and women to age 80. In the US and many other countries this average age extends years longer.

Centuries, even decades ago, people did not live long enough to develop dementia what with poor sanitation, little control of plagues and infectious diseases—to name just a few reasons. Even though today we are living longer, the environmental influence on our lives and our genetic makeup is precipitating what I believe to be near epidemic proportions of dementia.

It is estimated that fifty percent of people reaching age 82 will have some form of dementia. Alzheimer's disease being the most prevalent and prolific. This amounts to over 5 million people currently in the US. Not only is dementia a costly disease, requiring 24/7 care-giving, it consumes the lives of those suffering from this loss of mental cognition, and the family members who care for them.

Loss of cognitive function represents the number one fear among our senior population. As cognition decline ensues, so do motor skills and activities of daily living. Patients become frail, bed ridden, and often times combative and delusional.

Cognitive loss also causes physical and financial stress on family and care givers in equal measure. Alzheimer's is considered a *no option disease*. A disease for which we have little or no treatment.

I believe Alzheimer's disease can be preventable. A host of life-style factors that influence this disease such as stress, sleep, diet, exercise, vitamin and mineral deficiencies, and hormonal deficiencies are within your immediate grasp. In addition, social connections, family interactions and a purposeful life add important lifestyle factors. Avoiding toxic substances like heavy metals, chemicals and drugs (both prescription and street drugs) are critical. Avoiding genetically modified foods, a stressful lifestyle, making sure you eat organic clean food and having a pure water supply, are important to ensuring long-term health.

Any one of the above factors can facilitate inflammation in the central nervous system. By many indications these **causal associations** (cause and effect associations) seem to be a prerequisite to dementia formation. This book touches on some of these inflammatory casual associations, most of which are very complex. Entire books can be written the subject. I will attempt to present my years of experience and findings in laymen's terms for ease of reference and use.

Because dementia is a multi-factored problem it does not fit the typical **medical models**. Models that say, find the bacteria (infectious agent), discover a drug that will kill it, and we have a cure. This is what I call the "key in the lock" solution—one cause, one solution. Science has been looking for this *one* key . . . a drug, a monotherapy, a procedure that will remove the **tangles and plaque**—the invasive brain debris the medical community feels is the cause of Alzheimer's disease.

If we remove the tangles and plaque there is no guarantee such a procedure will help to restore memory. Medical science has a lot of nonagenarians who upon death were biopsied. They had a lot of tangles and plaque in their brains, yet had normal neurological function and memory at the time of their death.

Alzheimer's disease is not a simple cross word puzzle, no one "key" is the answer. Alzheimer's is a Rubik's Cube.

Alzheimer's and Epigenetics:
Epigenetics studies the effects of the environment on our genes. The subject of epigenetics needs to be addressed up-front as it will be referred to often by the various processes I write about. These are complex processes involved in the repair and reprogramming of the genetic structures within our cells.

The root word of epigenetics is "genetics". A term initially used to discuss the developmental evolution of mankind. Darwin and others established an "evolution of the species theory" which is still highly regarded by genetic scientists today. This theory states we are products of our genetic makeup. I intend to expand on this theory and address just a few of the environmental factors that are complicating our genetic development and hence our health from *in vivo*, natural fertilization, all the way to the grave.

Research continues to uncover dietary and environmental connections that affect not only the living but the unborn for generations to come. Once the genes are turned-on in human egg fertilization, there is no turning back. Our genetic makeup is set for life with this genetic code repeating itself in our offspring. As many may already know, scientific researchers sequenced the human **genome** using computer models. Genomes are the full DNA information needed to build and maintain your body. While the computer models helped medical scientists to understand *which* genes are *where,* for the most part we still do not understand what they *do.* We do not fully understand *how* they are expressed to determine individual make up.

Troubling events in the world in which we live have added a new dimension to this complex, but somewhat straight forward process of fertilization and normal development of a fetus, into a healthy viable birth. Events such as automation, industrialization, environmental control, or what we call progress, can often be a hindrance to good health even expediting this new study of epigenetics.

I will discuss in general about toxins, without going into detail about the mechanisms of how the toxins damage your neurological structures, but demonstrate the dire-strait facing human kind. In a study, the umbilical cord blood of babies was checked for environmental toxins. Of the 400 toxins checked, there were 256 positive results. The government calls this result "the toxic burden". I call it a crime.

In addition, the air pregnant women breathe was examined. It contained all of the toxins included in the original study. These toxins when aerosolized, including lead and mercury, accumulate in the body. A fetus' developing brain gets a heavier dose of toxins as the blood brain barrier is not yet developed. Thus, the dosage in the infant is much higher than in the adult.

California State recently passed legislation on requiring flame retardants be placed in mattresses—very toxic stuff for adults but a new mattress in the baby's room is disastrous for an infant's neural tissue. It is little wonder that fifteen percent of children born in the United States have a brain disability and that one in ninety boys are born on the autism spectrum.

Let me say without getting into a political diatribe; it appears that neither the government (EPA or FDA), nor big corporations care about your health—or giving you healthy products for daily living. One example is the fungicide Vinclozolin, used to control blights, rots and molds in vineyards, and on fruits and vegetables. Vinclozolin can affect DNA development within the cell causing cancer and kidney defects which are passed along to the fetus.

In another study, cocaine fed to mice passed on memory problems to descendants for three generations. Chronic methamphetamine use causes a Parkinsonion-like syndrome. Chronic alcoholism causes dementia and movement disorders. Even a small amount of alcohol can cause permanent damage to the developing brain of a fetus. I cannot imagine what we will eventually find with marijuana smokers since we know that marijuana affects the brain's consciousness and decision-making process.

Epigenetics is an exciting new field of study which will be with us for generations as we sort out the thousands of chemicals we are exposed to on a daily basis and their effects on the human body. Numerous studies have proven that "you are what you eat". Diet (even your mother's diet), can influence genes *in utero* and turn "on" or "off" genes depending on shortages or excesses of food processing and additives.

Parenting too, makes a difference as parental care is transferred to the child. Nervous or anxious mothers can pass this trait to their offspring.

Although not very practicable, the answer is to grow what you eat, avoid synthetic materials, food additives, pesticides . . . the list could go on and on. My advice is to read labels and try to eat organic wherever and whenever possible.

As you begin to read this book, you will find the changes you need to make are not that difficult. Most changes are common sense, but can require further research and some modest lifestyle changes to adapt to the suggestions made.

From this book I hope you will realize there are several likely "keys" to solving such a complex disease. The idea is, I want you to look at all the topics, one topic for each chapter. You can decide which subject or subjects are of most concern to you and go directly to them. **Bold** words within the text are further expounded on in a glossary in an appendix along with references highly recommended for further investigation on your own.

An action plan after each subject gives you some direction on how to go about resolving that topic. The nutritional supplements formulated by NutraGen™ are listed under the "Products" Chapter. There is no need to shop around for the right herb or supplement. The supplements have extensive research behind them, are sourced from the best organic products and formulated specifically to treat neurological diseases such as Alzheimer's disease.

I have had personal experience with Alzheimer's disease. My father-in-law lived with my wife and me in his final years. His story demonstrates just how invasive this disease can be. *Leo's Story* is my wife's heartfelt portrayal of our time shared together.

Leo's Story
By
Terry Woolley Howe

I grew up in what I consider to be a "vanilla" household. A two-parent, intact family where my parents devoted all of their free time to my two brothers and me. Mom became a Brownie and then a Girl Scout leader for me, and a Den Mother and Boy Scout leader for my brothers. She was president of the PTA, and my dad was the boys little league coach.

My parents were not very strict about most things, but my mother was a smoker and my dad did not want us to develop that habit. He explained to us, "If we wanted to smoke we should learn to do it with our feet because he would break both our arms." While he didn't mean it literally, he got his point across.

For my parent's 50th wedding anniversary, my brothers and I had a big party for them. Someone asked my dad what was the secret to staying married for 50 years. He said it was very simple, "You find the most perfect woman for you, and then you spend the next 50 years hiding the fact from her that she could have done better."

The smoking eventually caught up with my mom, and she developed COPD. After several years, my mom was not able to get out anymore and my dad became her caregiver. While we knew dad was getting forgetful, we assumed it was due to being sleep deprived. He simple would not let anyone else take care of my mom.

After 63 years of marriage, my mom passed in October, 2001. It was then that we came to realize dad suffered from dementia. Mom always handled the social calendar, paid bills, and organized everything. This so frequently happens in families where the spouse covers up the lapses in memory.

We were unaware of the severity of my dad's problem until mom was gone and dad was on his own. He probably had lived with memory problems for at least ten years. We asked if he wanted to live with us, but he said he had a house and wanted to live there. Every morning he would go to the YMCA and swim laps for half an hour then take a walk around the golf course.

I lived 150 miles from my dad, but it was not unusual for him to drive down for a few hours to visit and then drive home. But he started getting lost on the way home. So I began to take the train to his house on Thursday afternoon, spend the night and on Friday morning, we would drive back to our house for the weekend. I hoped that during the week, he was okay to be home alone. He was in his home town and in his own house that he had lived in for 60 years.

My brother stayed with him at night, Monday through Wednesday, but sometimes on the nights when my brother was not there, I would get calls from dad asking if his car was in the shop. He had driven some place for lunch, walked home and forgot where his car was. Or I would get a call from his *doctor because he had come to the office for an appointment. An appointment he did not have.*

When it became apparent that dad could no longer live alone, my brothers and I decided it would be best for him if he lived with me. It helped greatly that my husband was family oriented and also thought it best for my dad if he lived with us.

We told dad, he was going to stay with us for a while. He was okay with that. We never sold or modified his house. My dad and I would sometimes go there to stay, but after a day or two, he was happy to return to our home. We have a ranch away from the city with horses, dogs and cats. There was always something to do or see.

When dad first came to live with us, I tried to find projects for him to do to keep him busy. He had always liked refinishing furniture. We have an oak dining room table and I thought that would be a good project. We moved the table out onto the deck and he went to work sanding. When he had the sanding done to his satisfaction, he started putting on the varnish. He put on several layers and it was really looking great.

We were just waiting for it to completely dry so we could move it back inside. My mistake was going to the grocery store. When I got back, he had started sanding it again. He went through the entire process again.

When dad first came to live with us, he would do the New York Times crossword puzzle every morning. He also played solitaire. As time went on, we noticed him doing the crossword puzzles less and taking more naps in the rocking chair on the deck. We could see him slowing down and getting less involved in his surroundings. We realized we were on the slippery slope that happens for Alzheimer patients where they lose touch with their environment and lose their ability to take care of themselves.

My husband, David, was the Medical Director for Stemedica Cell Technologies, a stem cell company in San Diego, and had actually treated patients for stroke, spinal cord injury, and yes, even Alzheimer's disease. Stem cells were administered to help with his overall well-being along with the possibility of helping short term memory.

While the stem cells did not restore his short term memory, the treatment did give him a "new lease on life." He was back to doing the daily crossword puzzles, napping less and interacting with those around him. He continued to be active and feel physically well. He lived another four years and remained active.

I believe that the stem cell treatment dad received prevented him from lapsing into the moderate to final stages of Alzheimer's. He never experienced the moderate stages where some patients express poor judgment. He was not confused, and he didn't require help with activities of daily living. He picked out his own clothes to wear, dressed himself, showered, ate and was a pleasure to be around.

His personality never changed, which often happens to some Alzheimer patients. They become restless, agitated and sometimes, aggressive. Dad never developed any final stage symptoms, which happens to some patients where they lose the physical ability to walk or cannot control their bladder and bowels. I was able to care for my father without assistance until the day he peacefully died at our home in his bed.

I learned a lot from my dad throughout my life, and while taking care of him the last years of his life, I learned many things about caring for someone with Alzheimer's.

I learned to be patient. Things took longer and it didn't matter if he asked the same question ten times. I answered the question as if it was the first time, because for him, it was the first time.

I learned not to get my feelings hurt if he forgot something that I had told him that was important to me. I remember when I told my dad that our oldest daughter just had our first grandchild. He didn't remember it later. My initial thought was, "I can understand how you don't remember what you had for breakfast, but how could you not remember something so important as a grandchild?" Then I realized that he had no control over what was remembered. Whether it was what he had for breakfast, or whether there was a new grandchild, it was all gone in ten minutes.

I learned it wasn't necessary for me to go out of my way to do something extra special for him because he was not going to remember. It was important that the "now" be pleasant for him, because that was all there was.

I learned there was no anger history. If he got upset or impatient with me when I was busy trying to finish something, in ten minutes that anger was gone – the slate wiped clean.

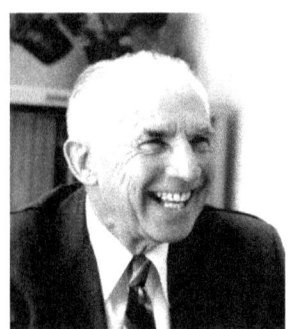

Leo Rollans

I learned if he was going to do a project of refinishing furniture, that when he got to the varnish stage, I needed to hide the sandpaper.

PART ONE

Consequence

Alzheimer's Disease

Alzheimer's is a disease of the brain. Diagnosis is difficult in the initial stages because the brain has such great **reserve capacity** *of coping capabilities. Medical practitioner's estimate, once a diagnosis is determined, the patient has undergone neurological damage for approximately ten years.*

People often ask me, "What is the difference between dementia and Alzheimer's?" The word dementia in recent decades has taken the place of an older term, senility. Today dementia denotes a symptom for which there are many causes.

To give an analogy; if we said the patient had a fever, we would recognize it as a symptom for which there are many problems. The fever does not tell us the problem or underlying cause, only that there is one. Similarly dementia does not tell us the problem only that there is one with Alzheimer's disease being the most common.

As you read through this book, you will recognize several causal (cause and effect) etiologies for dementia. Medical literature frequently refers to any deficit in cognitive function as Alzheimer's. It really is important to eliminate all other possible causes of dementia with thorough testing.

Pathology studies estimate that thirty percent of Alzheimer's diagnosis have a vascular (blood vessel) underlying factor. **Vascular dementia** can be a primary etiology, or result from a secondary complicating factor. For example: Mild cognitive impairment (MCI), is a primary etiology that can be complicated by secondary hypertension, diabetes, or heart disease factors. These secondary factors often times accelerate the progression of MCI into full blown Alzheimer's disease. Alcoholism and hypothyroidism are also high on the list as recognized causes of dementia.

As we age, it is normal to lose brain volume. **Mentation**, our thought processes, often slow down right alongside our physical function. There are some newer imaging technologies like **Magnetic resonance imaging (MRI)** although helpful, they do not give a definitive diagnostic tool for Alzheimer's disease. In addition, there are no blood tests to make it easier for doctors to make a diagnosis of Alzheimer's disease.

The test doctors commonly turn to in order to determine if cognitive impairment is indeed Alzheimer's is called the Mini-Mental State Examination (MMSE) test. This test involves monitoring answers to 30 questions that fit into six different categories: registration, attention, calculation, recall, language, and orientation. Once the test is taken, an algorithm score is assigned the patient. Depending on the number of correct answers, the tester can evaluate if the dementia is mild, moderate or severe.

The tests are mostly paper and pencil, where the doctor asks the patient a series of questions and records their answers. The questions are usually about current events, such as:

- Who is the president of the United States?

- Who is your senator?

- What day is it today?

There are also some math questions like, "Count backwards from 96 subtracting 7 each time." This gives the evaluator a very good idea of the patient's connection with reality. You can go to the following website and download a test to take on your own:

www.alzheimersreadingroom.com/p/test-your-memory-for-alzheimers-5-best.html

There are stages each patient will go through, beginning with MCI to advanced disease. The scales differ but are frequently divided into 5 or 7 stages. At the beginning, patients may recognize their short term memory loss. This is not a simple misplacing of your keys—if it were, my wife would have been institutionalized 30 years ago! This is, "I cannot recall what I had for dinner tonight." one hour after a meal. Such short term memory gradually worsens in severity until eventually you may have a patient who is non-functional, bed ridden, incontinent and in diapers, becoming angry and/or frustrated. Frequently, they must be institutionalized because they are combative, at times abusive, and completely unaware of their disconnect with reality.

Patients in the moderate to severe classification need constant supervision. They may drive the car someplace and forget how to get home. They forget to turn off the stove, or they will wander off in the store or the neighborhood and forget where they are. My father-in-law would call us in the early morning and want to know if his car was in the auto repair shop. When in actuality he forgot where he parked it the afternoon before and had simply walked home.

This can be a dangerous stage for activities like driving. They should have the car keys taken away and told that they do not have a driver's license.

3

I have found it very interesting, how patients with moderate Alzheimer's can carry on a conversation with a stranger for quite some time and the stranger never recognizes that there is a problem. This is because they are using knowledge previously programmed in their memory bank and not current knowledge.

I frequently get asked to give a prognosis as to how long the patient will live considering their current condition. There was a long term study performed by Baylor University on this very subject. Patients were divided into 3 groups: fast progression, moderate progression, and slow progression. A number of factors were used in the evaluation and patients were placed into one of the above-mentioned three groups. Several tests were administered and recorded over the patient's lifetime. Patient survival in the rapidly progressing group was 2½ years and in the slow group an average of 5 years. Other studies report that the average survival is about 8 years from the time of diagnosis.

When patients first begin showing signs of dementia, the symptoms are usually vague. The spouse frequently recognizes the memory loss first and sometimes covers up this memory malfunction to family and friends out of embarrassment. So even some loved ones are unaware for a period of time. The patient themselves are frequently in denial about the severity of their problem.

I am familiar with the challenges of Alzheimer's, having lived with someone who succumbed to the disease. I liken it to existing in physical form only and sometimes being detached from reality. When one is cognitively not present, there is little purpose in life.

There are currently 24 million people in the world who have a diagnosis of Alzheimer's disease. As the world population ages, and with the increase in longevity, this number is expected to double by 2040. The cost of this disease is only a guess because caregiver hours are often provided by families.

Alzheimer's disease is associated with aging, where it is estimated that 50% of the people who live to be 82 years of age will suffer from Alzheimer's or other forms of dementia. The disease now affects one in nine persons older than 65 years of age. It is expected to increase in the United States by 40%, affecting over 7 million Americans by 2025.

Alzheimer's disease has many of the same possible etiologies/pathologies as traumatic brain injury, Parkinson's, multiple sclerosis (MS), and amyotrophic lateral sclerosis (ALS) or sometimes known as Lou Gehrig's disease. A look at the brain under the microscope upon autopsy shows many similarities.

Clinically, these diseases have recognized shorter life spans. Parkinson's patients die on average 6 years after diagnosis, ALS 42 months after diagnosis. Alzheimer's disease death rates vary with the 'rapidly progressive diagnoses' at only 2½ years and the 'slowly progressive' 5 to 8 years after diagnosis. Each of these diseases may well affect specific portions of the brain more notably than other parts, but eventually they all affect the entire brain.

All of these conditions cause depression, dementia, balance problems, movement disorders, slowing of mentation, and autonomic dysfunction (bladder and bowel control). Of these deteriorations, all interfere with a patient's ability to function both cognitively and physically. Because of these similarities, when testing for any of these neurological diseases, we look for heavy metals, toxic chemicals, infectious agents, metabolic abnormalities, vitamin and hormonal deficiencies, and drug toxicities as possible causal etiologies.

Action Plan:
In the following chapters we will discuss what action is needed to address the possible multiple causes of Alzheimer's. Also in the back of this book under Part 5. Here you will find a full action plan showing how to get started and a listing on how to go about addressing the causes. There is also information about the NutraGen™ product line that can be most beneficial. I highly recommend this product be taken no matter your age or condition.

There are a few newer imaging technologies that can determine buildup of **amyloid plaque** (incorrectly folded protein fragment). Positron emission tomography (PET) scans now use a special contrast injection which will show heavy concentration of amyloid in the brain. Also new and less invasive is an eye imaging device which uses high-tech lenses to take a picture of the eye to diagnose amyloid build up.

Diabetes

Alzheimer's, long believed to be closely related to diabetes disease, is frequently referred to in medical circles as "type III diabetes".

If you have type II diabetes, your liver is producing **amyloid**, an abnormal protein most commonly produced in bone marrow. This is the same amyloid that produces tangle and plaques in the brain of Alzheimer's patients and labeled type III diabetes.

With diabetes, the muscle cells develop insulin resistance, a condition in which the body produces insulin but does not use it effectively. This is a metabolic problem recognized early in the disease and worsens with its severity.

The neural cells in the brain also develop insulin resistance which worsens as Alzheimer's progresses. We consider the **endothelial tissue** as having the first changes that occur in this **metabolic syndrome**. Metabolic syndrome is a cluster of conditions signaling the very beginning of diabetes, such as:

- Hypertension
- Endothelial dysfunction
- Obesity
- Cardiac conditions

What patients neglect to recognize is that these changes do not happen in isolation. If, for example, the blood vessels of the heart are plugged up, then the blood vessels elsewhere are also affected. The liver and lower extremities will be compromised and the brain will exhibit **vascular dementia**.

Diabetes is frequently associated with obesity and cardiovascular disease. This triad of diseases demonstrates a multitude of hormonal, metabolic and vascular pathology affecting the whole body, and needs to be addressed as part of an overall comprehensive treatment program. It is important to mention here a definite link between diabetes and dihydroepiandosterone (DHEA), an adrenal hormone.

DHEA, the most abundant steroid hormone in the blood, is produced mostly by the adrenal gland. A low level of DHEA has shown to be an early marker for diabetes. What role DHEA plays in the metabolic cycle is still in question. A precursor hormone to testosterone and estrogens, DHEA becomes an important player in the steroid hormone cycle. In my opinion, it needs to be supplemented to a healthy range in order to have effective diabetes treatment.

Researchers have found if a nasal insulin preparation is administered, this allows insulin to get into the brain and slow down the decline of cognitive function. This procedure reinforces the theory that Alzheimer's disease is indeed part and parcel of the systemic disease known as type II diabetes.

Action Plan:
Make certain that you get a workup for diabetes, including: blood pressure, HbA1c, fasting insulin levels, triglycerides, basal metabolic index, and tests for inflammatory mediators like

fibrinogen, homocysteine, hsCRP thyroid hormone panel, and Endothelian-1.

From these tests, the severity of the diabetes can be determined as well as the amount of inflammation in your body. Other tests of interest would be a lipid panel, ECG, weight measurement and echo cardiogram. These will give a good baseline to measure against.

News releases recently out of Austria indicate that a high fat diet normalizes blood sugar levels and is beneficial in type II diabetes. Blood sugar, triglycerides, obesity, blood pressure, are all considered important indicators of metabolic syndrome which is also referred to as pre-diabetes. Regardless of what you call it, pre-diabetes is the beginning of a progressive disease which affects the entire body.

There is suggested reading in the appendix of this book which explains what I refer to as the optimal "paleo type" diet. The general concept is to eat more fats and proteins, and less refined carbohydrates. The percentages of intake should be as follows:

- 40-50% fat

- 30% protein

- 20-30% complex carbohydrates

This is very different from the usual dietary recommendations of the American Diabetic Association and the American Heart Association.

Remember, these are two groups that have encouraged the American people to eat the Standard American Diet (SAD) which resulted in record numbers of diabetics, and caused heart disease to be the number-one cause of death in the United States. Read *Blood Sugar Solution* by Mark Hyman, M.D. It lays out an excellent plan to put you back on the correct dietary pathway.

You need to lose weight to optimal basal metabolic index (BMI) as your stored body fat secretes numerous inflammatory factors and cytokines. Remember inflammation is the hallmark of neuro-degenerative diseases.

Incorporate the nutritional products outlined in this book and follow a paleo diet. Find a doctor that will help you do this. Help is available. If you cannot find help, follow the suggestions in this book and do it yourself.

Brain Injury

There is a plethora of news media reports and expert opinion on the eventual outcome of head trauma leading to dementia and ultimately Alzheimer's disease.

Traumatic brain injury (TBI) is a well-recognized causal etiology for dementia. Such is evidenced by the increased incidents found in professional football players who have had repeated concussions.

We know from the news that football players have an increased incidence of neurological disease including dementia. The incidence is highest amongst the "big guys". Although they all are mostly big, I am talking about the players on the offensive and defensive lines, the linemen.

Do they suffer because they have multiple head traumas from fighting in the trenches where each play may cause bruising damage to the brain tissue . . .

- or is it because they are so overly fat (the wrong type of fat which is loaded with inflammatory factors) and have metabolic syndrome/diabetes?

- or to keep the extra pounds on they eat more genetically modified foods and high carbohydrate diets?

- or is the issue because they are exposed to more Lyme tick **antigen** in the grass, weed killer poison on the grass, along with the synthetic turf?

- or because of their size *do* football players require additional vital nutrients? Are they not getting enough of the nutrients as mentioned in this book?

- or does possible brain trauma *set the stage* and the other factors complicate matters to allow neuro-degenerative diseases to develop?

The question is . . . is it all of the above or two or more of the above causal etiologies? Which is it?

Unfortunately, such associations are not so simple. Some of the pathology may take years to develop. And often, a TBI is caused by repeated exposures, or the disease is precipitated by one event.

In fact, not until a few years ago did many Americans become aware of severe head trauma **sequelae**. Even minor but repeated head trauma can also be dangerous and cause dementia.

As I write this, the National Football League has authorized payment for treatment of former players who suffer head trauma in their football careers. They call this chronic traumatic encephalopathy (CTE) and presents itself as:

- Dementia

- Alzheimer's

- ALS

- Parkinson's disease

- Migraine headache

- Seizure disorders

- Depression

Along with other diseases that show up later as we see the sequelae, the aftermath of conditions associated with the damaged neurons, as a head injury unfolds.

NFL players have a fourfold increase in Alzheimer's disease. A new study found that three out of ten NFL players will develop Alzheimer's disease at a much earlier time in life and double the frequency of the general population.

In this study, it was determined that 28% of the players in the league would develop Alzheimer's, moderate dementia or other serious neurological conditions like ALS or Parkinson's. There are 19,000 former players living which mean that 6,000 of them will be victims of traumatic brain injury. Most of the studies use statistics of 5 years playing in the league to qualify for the study.

We know that just one TBI (this does not include open skull fracture) can cause serious brain trauma and result in Alzheimer's disease and dementia. So the numbers here are huge. This is not to mention the military veterans who are coming home from foreign conflict with brain trauma from improvised explosive device (IED) explosions. I believe these numbers dwarf the NFL numbers. By far the most significant number of TBI's come from:

- Automobile accidents

- Sporting accidents

- Slip and fall accidents

We regretfully have no accepted therapy for these injuries—either to halt their progression or to repair and regenerate the damaged neurological tissue. Could it be that many of the violent crimes that are committed are because of previously unrecognized head trauma affecting the impulse control centers.

Action Plan:
You should not, nor should you allow your children, to play sports without protective head gear. This means any sport that can cause injury to the head such as off road bikes, off track motorized 2 and 4 wheeled vehicles, football, hockey and rugby. And the list goes on.

Absolutely no boxing or contact martial arts participation is recommended. Even "heading" the ball in soccer is a really bad idea, especially girls, as their muscle and ligamentous structures are different than boys. Girls' neck structures are not as stable.

In my opinion, with any of these sports, it is not a matter of *if* there will be an injury, but merely a matter of *when.*

We now have neurological testing to determine TBI's. This testing is noninvasive and measures the brain waves of the brain. Sequential testing can be done to determine if the brain is healing or has healed itself sufficiently to return to play after a sports injury. There are several states that have "Return to Learn" laws that govern educational learning assessment after brain trauma.

There is however no treatment for brain injury outside of acute care and rest. If symptoms persist I recommend a nutritional support system should be instituted as described in Part Five, Getting Started.

I just assisted in writing a stem cell protocol for TBI's. If you suffer from persistent symptoms of TBI, keep abreast of the stem cell research currently under way. Refer to Part Three, Neural Regulation and Repair, and Stem Cells.

—NOTES—

PART TWO

Environmental Perpetrators

Anesthesia

Frequently we are not aware of certain activities being dangerous such as anesthesia administered for pain before a surgical procedure.

Although few people ever read the disclaimer before a surgical procedure, it is a scary document. Usually, the doctor states they are going to put you to sleep, or something similar. If he said, "We are going to place you into a coma." most people would panic and have second thoughts. However, a coma is the best description for what is happening.

For children under age 3, general anesthesia can result in *Attention Deficit Disorder*, learning disabilities, and in 73% of cases, problems with abstract thinking. These issues are no doubt the effect of general anesthetics on the developing brain.

Doctors and researchers first learned of this problem in adults after prolonged open heart surgeries. Patients and after surgery caregivers found there was significant cognitive decline of memory loss, mental fog, and an inability to concentrate. Often full brain function never returned to pre-surgical level.

As we age, there are fewer neurotransmitter substances in the brain. General anesthesia lowers these neurotransmitter levels enough to cause memory problems and cognitive decline.

Over the years in my medical practice, I have had numerous patients with neuro-degenerative disease like Parkinson's or dementia. They tell me the general anesthesia they had for a knee replacement or heart surgery was the turning point in their health. Their disease, the onset of ALS, Parkinson's or Alzheimer's, was brought on by the anesthetic they received for surgery.

In addition, studies show that seniors receive too much anesthetic during procedures. This can lead to complications not only during surgery but also during the surgical recovery phase. Ask for just enough *sleep* to get the surgery performed.

All anesthetics have side effects and should not be considered safe. Their effects can be felt for weeks, months, even for a lifetime. There are 60,000 surgeries done in the U.S. daily, but know that a *routine procedure* could have lifelong consequences. If surgery is in your future, please talk to your doctor about what anesthetic is going to be used.

Famous comedian and talk show host, Joan Rivers, at age 81, underwent a minor surgery. During the surgical procedure she went into cardiac arrest and ended up hospitalized in intensive care. Her heart stopped and she became unresponsive. How many brain cells did she lose during the time her brain was deprived of oxygen? Joan died a week later. One has to ask, If she had survived, would she have ever been the same, mentally or physically?"

Action Plan:
Unfortunately, the best advice I have is to avoid general anesthesia at all costs after age 50. For some surgeries, a spinal anesthetic or conscious sedation is possible.

A face lift to remove a few facial wrinkles may be a decision very costly to your health. If you have no choice, please follow the plan I have outlined in the back of this book to increase your neurotransmitter count prior to, during, and post-surgery. This will help to minimize the effects of the anesthetic. Take the protein powder and B complex vitamin to ensure you have the raw materials to make new neurotransmitters. In addition, the antioxidants will help you detox the anesthetics.

—NOTES—

Drugs – Legal or Otherwise

Street drugs are dangerous enough but legal prescription drugs can be dangerous too.

Drugs, like the ever-popular statin drugs (a class of drugs prescribed to lower blood cholesterol) are all linked to dementia and cataracts. In animal models where statin drugs were administered, cognitive function problems became profound. Several statin drugs are:

- Lipitor

- Zocor

- Lescol

- Pravachol

- Crestor

I believe a recent association between statin drugs and ALS has been recognized by doctors but is being silenced by the pharmaceutical industry.

Such cognitive complications are addressed in the fine print on all drug package inserts but usually never relayed to the patient as possible side effects. All antipsychotic drugs are neurotoxin meaning they directly affect our nervous system, such as:

- Sleeping pills

- Painkillers

- Anti-anxiety drugs

- Cholesterol drugs

- Incontinence drugs

- Acid reflux (proton pump inhibitors)

- Blood pressure drugs

- Tranquilizers

- Heart drugs

- Anti-Parkinson's drugs

It is estimated that 15-30% of patients diagnosed with Alzheimer's disease have been misdiagnosed due to adverse or drug interactions as a causal etiology for their dementia. If you are taking more than three different prescription drugs, they are working against each other and causing you more harm than good.

Tell your doctor that you do not want to take unnecessary medications. It is of vital importance to avoid all drugs that either are not necessary or do not work. You should only take those necessary to keep you alive. Eliminate all others.

Legal prescription drugs can be dangerous enough but street drugs most assuredly are. Methamphetamines, heroin, and other mind-expanding drugs such as LSD may have long-term effect, even if only used once.

Cocaine administered to rats (rats are considered by researchers as a legitimate model for this research) affected the DNA methylation process in the brain for at least 3 generations—

methylation process being a significant step in the development of neurological tissue. Without methylation, we cannot make new DNA or repair DNA in the body.

Only one in ten prescription drug interaction or drug related complications are reported to authorities. Yet drug complications are the leading cause of hospitalizations. There would likely be a revolution if even half were reported.

Yale University research indicated that twenty percent of all hospital discharges are re-admitted to the hospital within thirty days because of medication complications. This re-admission rate does not bode well for our hospital system whose doctors are known for loading patients up on drugs before they leave. Sometimes asking a caring pharmacist is best, as they know the drugs and drug interactions better than physicians.

The FDA just lowered the recommended dosage of Tylenol dramatically. Tylenol has been found to cause liver and kidney failure, and reportedly responsible for 68,000 hospital visits per year.

A recent article in the news reported new research revealing the popular drug group benzodiazepines, of which valium is best recognized, are a cause of dementia. Benzodiazepine is a family of minor tranquilizers. Over the past forty years, doctors have used this group of drugs for a number of things:

- Anxiety
- Muscle relaxants
- Sleeping aids

The uses are really too numerous to mention them all. And all are used without knowing they cause brain damage and likely doing more harm than good.

Action Plan:
Get off any drugs that you do not absolutely need to be on to stay alive. Even pills like baby aspirin to keep your blood from clotting.

I have found taking baby aspirin to thin your blood has not been effective. The benefits do not outweigh the detriments, as it causes stomach bleeds and is a frequent cause of hospitalizations as we age.

Statin drugs, which may help a very small hereditary hypercholesterolemia group, are of questionable help as they are known to contribute to dementia. Any opioid type drug including: codeine, hydrocodone, and all of the morphine associated drugs for pain, should be avoided.

These drugs all alter your mental state and contribute to dementia. Be careful of the benzodiazepines mentioned above and other "sleeping aids" including Benadryl.

Take your drugs to the pharmacist and ask him/her about drug-to-drug adverse interactions. Your pharmacist can do a computer search that will give you the answers you need about dangerous adverse effects of drug combinations.

Household Chemicals

Chemical toxicity is not limited to industrial emissions and manufacturing facilities. Chemical toxicity can be found invading our lives right in our own homes.

Benzene, a natural component of crude oil and gasoline, provides the sweet smell in the air at the gas pump. It is a solvent used to make **phthalates**. Phthalates are the substance added to plastics to increase their flexibility, transparency, durability, and longevity. There are millions of gallons made of this every year. Benzene and plastics have invaded our lives.

Phthalates are also hormone disruptors and have an adverse effect on the thyroid hormone as well as male and female hormones. They shed off the plastics containers, plates, eating utensils into our drinking water, sodas, juice, milk… the list can go on and on. If the plastic is heated in the microwave, phthalates shed even more.

Plastics are widely used often without our even being fully conscious of their presence. Many foods are sold in plastic containers along with aluminum cans, most notably beverage cans, coated in bisphenol (BPA) secreting plastics.

These plastics are known endocrine disruptors along with rubber, and other synthetic materials which again shed toxic substances like BPA and polyvinyl chlorides (PVC's). Both toxins being carcinogenic when inhaled, or neurotoxic when ingested. Plastics can be found in:

- Vinyl flooring
- Children's backpacks
- Building materials
- Personal care products

To name just a few.

There are plastics that do not shed phthalates. They are more costly to produce. But you should use them if you are drinking out of sports bottles or using baby bottles.

Use glass bottles if at all possible.

In addition, people who have been employed where they were exposed to benzene, chlorinated solvents, and petroleum solvents are predisposed to cancer and neurological diseases. Research has linked workers in these industries with chemical exposures to early dementia, memory and critical thinking problems. Chemical solvents are very toxic and are found in:

- Paints
- Glues
- Degreasers
- Aerosolized sprays
- Cigarette smoke

Yes, cigarette smoke is another source of benzene exposure.

Other chemicals, like insect repellant, fungicide for plant and weed killers (like *Round Up*) are all neurotoxines and have been implicated as causal etiologies for Parkinson's and Alzheimer's diseases.

Vinclozlin, a fungicide found in weed killer and fertilizers for your grass and used on the vegetables and fruits found in your grocery store, causes neurological damage, cancer and kidney defects. It too, has a profound negative effect on reproductive and hormone systems affecting DNA genetics for future generations. Contact with these chemicals are to be avoided at all costs.

Often times, one is not aware of the dangers. One of my patients had exposure to a Paraquat insecticide spray which he used on his roses. Over a period of years he had regular exposure with this chemical. Both he and his neurologist blamed his Parkinson's disease on this regular exposure to such a neurotoxic substance.

On our ranch, we recently began a planting program of bougainvillea plant vines which of course, attracted insects. I had to really look for products with natural ingredients to rid the plants of the invading pests as most of the products on the market contain a host of toxic chemicals which we cannot pronounce, let alone know the toxic effects associated with their use.

Action Plan:
Read the labels and stay away from all toxic sprays. To give a recent example of the problem, the other morning I awoke to some unfamiliar smells. Overnight, our kitchen had an ant invasion. This is not unusual as we live in the country where ants are large in number. Upon inspection, there were a host of dead ants. I asked my wife how she killed the ants. The aerosol spray she used, I found, was a neurotoxin spray.

As humans inhale this spray, what does it do to the nervous system? The end result cannot be good. I am sure the chemical company that makes this product has done dose-escalation studies to find what level of exposure can create symptoms in humans. But did they perform these studies on infants and people who are ages 70 to 80 on the edge of neurological impairment?

You should stay away from aerosol sprays. There are organic options, so read the labels. Do not trust the Environmental Protection Agency (EPA) and the USFDA as they are in business to protect the chemical industry, not you the consumer. Look for products that use plastics which do not shed BPA, PVC's or Phthalates. And remember to wash fruit and vegetables before eating. Preferably with an organic product free of chemicals.

This is a big subject, too comprehensive to cover here. But you should look for natural products and perform a little research, as this could prolong or even save your brain function. It should be noted that the State of California requires physicians to report any suspected cases of pesticide poisoning to State agencies.

Toxic Metals

Toxic metal exposure is an ongoing daily problem. Lead, cadmium, mercury and arsenic are in our daily food supply.

Metals are very toxic, not only for your brain, but for all of your other organs as well. Not long ago, I was reading that arsenic levels in our bodies are quite high. Of course, like you, I questioned. "How am I exposed to this toxin?"

It turns out that many of the Southern American cotton fields were sprayed with pesticides that contained arsenic, and the acreage is now being used to grow rice. The arsenic is still in the soil in high concentrations from years of spraying cotton plants with pesticides containing arsenic. Arsenic, which has an affinity for rice plants, is taken up in the rice kernels and when eaten, creates arsenic poisoning in our bodies.

Mercury comes from ingestion of fish. Almost all fish from the sea now contain mercury. Previously I could depend on Alaskan or Norwegian harvested fish to be free of heavy metals, but no longer, as the entire ocean is now contaminated.

Mercury and other toxic metals come from coal-burning power plants. The Chinese have thousands of these power plants and the aerosolized metals float in a jet stream right over to the United States.

The high pollution index is so alarming in China that lung disease is now the number one cause of death. The pollution index from our government, states that under 25ppm (parts per million) is generally recognized as safe. In Beijing, this count is routinely over 250 ppm and occasionally gets over 500 ppm. If the particle count is high, you know that the aerosolized pollutants will also be high. If you have lung or heart disease, it is important that you stay indoors during those days when the count is high.

As an example to demonstrate the toxicity of just *one* of these metals. A Harvard University epidemiologist who spoke at a conference I attended, stated that they could measure the amount of lead in a pregnant woman's upper arm (humorous bone) and from this measurement of lead content, could predict the IQ of her baby. Now this information is scary and one can imagine how neurotoxic lead is… and our bodies are often *filled* with this metal.

Aluminum too, is a toxic metal often implicated in Alzheimer's. I believe it is a major factor in Alzheimer's as it is so abundant in our diet and daily lives. To name just a few, there are many more:

- Aluminum cookware

- Soda cans

- Aluminum foil

There has been a renewed awareness of problems with the drinking water in many of America's cities. This broke in the news in a big way with the contamination of the drinking water in Michigan cities. The problem is so bad an immediate solution is not possible. This has led to a close examination of the water in many cities across the country. An environmental company called Environmental Working Group (EWG) has sounded the alarm about this pollution.

EWG just released a groundbreaking new analysis showing the notorious "Erin Brockovich" carcinogen, otherwise known as chromium-6, contaminates the tap water of two-thirds of Americans at levels above those scientists deem safe. The EWG website (www.ewg.org) is well worth checking out for numerous articles on health concerns.

Action Plan:
The "toxic metals" load can be measured within your body by using an EDTA challenge test. This test can be administered by an alternative medicine doctor who has knowledge of heavy metal burden. Lead, mercury, aluminum, arsenic and the other 17 toxic metals are all neurotoxic and the levels can be measured using this test.

NOTE: if your doctor wishes to check these levels with just a blood test, this will not be accurate and likely be negative.

I believe that any single toxic metal (and most of us have *several* toxic metals in high concentrations in our bodies) can be a causal etiology of Alzheimer's disease, so it is important that you get your levels measured. If they are high you should have them chelated out by an alternative medicine doctor who performs this procedure.

Oral chelating agents are available to rid the body of mercury, lead and other toxic metals. I use both intravenous treatment as well as oral chelation to rid the body of toxic metals.

Eliminate aluminum cookware, aluminum cans, and plastics as they shed phthalates, and all **haloids** (bromium, chlorine and fluoride). Have a home water filter installed to filter out chlorine, fluoride and toxic metals found in public water systems.

Begin the nutritional supplements listed at the end of this book. These will help the liver detox your system and help to rebuild both your metabolic and neurological structures.

PART THREE

Underlying Factors that Set the Stage

Hormones

There is a strong relationship between age-related loss of testosterone and estrogen to brain health.

When I use the word hormones, women think of estrogen and men think of testosterone. These are important for your health because when they are at low levels, vibrancy is also low. Since both men and women possess both of these hormones, when these two hormones are balanced, they make a remarkable difference in the well-being of the patient.

After 40 years in practice, I've found that both men and women feel and think better when these hormones are balanced and brought back into a healthy range. Hormones like progesterone are also very important as they act as neurotransmitters in the brain.

In the news today, it was reported that doctors found low testosterone and high estrogen in men as being predictive of a heart attack. This frequently occurs in older men, and men who have high body fat. Testosterone determines how hard the heart can beat and is an important hormone for heart health. These steroid hormones when in balance appear to have a protective effect on brain health as well.

Another hormone playing a major function in the brain is the thyroid hormone. Many medical professionals think the thyroid hormone is a major factor in Alzheimer's disease and dementia.

It turns out that toxins, like bromine used in bread and pastries, and fluoride added to the water supply and tooth paste along with chlorine found in the water you drink, were all placed there gradually, over time and supposedly, to protect us. We now know that they do just the opposite as they are toxic haloids, foreign and toxic to the thyroid and brain tissue. In fact, bromide, chlorine, and fluoride are all toxic. Together they are a disaster imperiling the health of millions of unsuspecting Americans who are under the false impression that the environmental protection agency (EPA) and the food and drug administration (FDA) are protecting the American public.

These bad haloid toxins interfere with iodine on the thyroid molecule to create hypothyroid disease. We know that pregnant women who are hypothyroid and their babies born with hypothyroidism are mentally delayed. The thyroid has a profound influence on brain health, and needs special attention in Alzheimer's disease.

If a patient with dementia has low thyroid, the problem may be greatly improved or even cured if the thyroid hormone is balanced and brought into the normal laboratory range.

Action Plan:
In my practice, I use a combination thyroid medication like "Armors Thyroid" or "Nature Thyroid" – these contain both types of thyroid necessary to return your metabolism to proper function.

Seek an alternative medicine doctor who appreciates and is knowledgeable on balancing thyroid hormone. The thyroid, adrenals and pancreas all have energy-producing hormones.

A comprehensive exam should also include a Reverse T3 lab test. This will measure an inert form of thyroid hormone created by toxic haloids: fluorine, chlorine, and bromine as mentioned above. These haloids are to be avoided at all costs as they are hormone disruptors.

These haloids are difficult to eliminate as they are so pervasive in our environment and food supply. One has to work at it at first, but soon you will be buying toothpaste without fluoride, filtering your tap water to eliminate chlorine, getting your swimming pool treated with ozone and making or seeking bread without GMO grains and bromine.

In order to balance the steroid hormones properly you need to do an entire panel of hormones and balance them all. I prescribe what are called "bioidentical hormones". These are made from yam and soy, and are not synthetic. They are identical to the hormones that are normally secreted by your body. Unlike the synthetic hormones, these are processed by the body's normal functions and do not build up to toxic levels in the body as the synthetics do.

Remember hormones are the master control molecules and need to be balanced not only for skin health but also to maintain great cognitive function.

The Environmental Working Group (EWG) website has as its tag statement "Know your Environment. Protect your Health". EWG addresses how the environment impacts an individual's well-being with such topics as what's in your tap water, shampoo, cleaners, pesticides, and on your food? What are GMOs? What do they do to our land and water—and many more topics related to hormones and our health in general. This is a good site to keep on your list for informative articles relating to your health and the environment you live in. The website is www.ewg.org and has a private search engine for articles such as the "Dirty Dozen Endocrine Disruptors" listing some prevalent toxins to our body's hormone balance.

Vitamin D

Vitamin D is really a hormone.

Vitamin D is converted from cholesterol to vitamin D on the surface of the skin in the presence of sunlight. This requires *direct* exposure of the skin *without* sun screen and clothing. There have been thousands of articles written on vitamin D, indicating it's involvement in bone formation, immune system function, and maintenance of cognitive function. Just to name a few functions.

It is thought that vitamin D influences the **microglia** (immune system cells) of the brain to remove the plaques. Even in areas like the American South, Southwest desert states and Southern California, where there is more sun exposure, there is an astounding deficiency of vitamin D in the populace.

Vitamin D deficiency is prevalent in Europe and Asia as well. This problem is very evident in China where the women cherish white skin. They not only use whiteners on their skin, but cover their faces and use umbrellas in the summertime to block the sun which would stimulate melanin and give them an undesirable tan. It also gives them an undesirable vitamin D deficiency which has a systemic effect on their health.

In seniors, the effect of the Vitamin D deficiency in cognitive performance is four times greater than in their younger cohorts.

41

The medical community has overlooked this hormone as a cause of muscle weakness and fragility in seniors far too long.

Just a few short years ago, the recommended dose for vitamin D was 400 IU's per day. Today, many believe that 2000-4000 IU should be the recommended dose.

A flood of information this past year concerning vitamin D as a substance that enhances cognitive function and overall brain health has finally sprung forth. Vitamin D is finally getting the attention it deserves. The Mayo clinic just published a paper which drew a direct connection between vitamin D levels and early mortality.

Action Plan:
It is easy to measure and treat this hormone deficiency by having a simple blood test to determine your levels.

Supplementing vitamin D and getting more sun exposure, along with fresh fruits and vegetables, usually brings vitamin D levels into the normal range.

Most doctors think that levels in the upper end of the normal range are best and will make for better bones and a happier brain.

The Mouth as a Source of Infection

It is an unfortunate shortsightedness of medicine that we overlook the mouth as a source of chronic disease. It is one area that can quickly become a sewer—a reservoir of disease for the whole body.

Unfortunately, the mouth is a difficult area to address because dental procedures like the following enhance the expansion of infection-causing bacteria:

- Amalgam fillings
- Root canals, crown and bridges
- Dental implants and titanium posts
- Cadaver implants for the jaw
- Veneer covers

These processes allow the multitude of bugs in our mouth to gain access and are all implicated in the erosion of the gums and bone, adding to the pockets that enhance the expansion of infection-causing bacteria. All are bacterial havens for the teeth. All cosmetic procedures contribute nothing towards a healthy mouth.

I also believe some of the problem is the overuse of antibiotics. The fact is we live longer and are prone to gingivitis and bone deterioration caused from poor circulation and vitamin D deficiency.

43

You hear dentists talk about plaque and flossing as a way to keep the mouth cleaner. What they are suggesting is bacteria form's a biofilm and can hide from the natural defense mechanisms of the body. I treat the mouth and its bacteria conditions by having the dentist use a laser to remove the plaque (biofilm) on the teeth. This limits the pockets where mycoplasma, **spirochetes** and other bacteria multiply.

Foreign materials like mercury **haptens.** Haptens are small molecules which cause autoimmune disease. It is a scientific fact that toxic metals like mercury are found in amalgam and even synthetic dental fillings. Even though we know these fillings contain mercury they are continued to be used by some dentists. Mercury is neurotoxic and is implicated in Alzheimer's disease.

The government warns people about eating too much sea food containing mercury, but also should warn about mercury products used in dentistry. My advice is to seek a biological dentist who can safely remove the amalgam fillings and crowns that contain amalgam. Verify that the dentist has the newest synthetic material being used to fill your teeth, and be tested to make sure that you not are allergic to it.

At all cost, avoid titanium/amalgam implants, root canals, and cadaver bone implants. A few dentists (Dr. Hal Huggins, Dr. Boyd Haley, Dr. Mercola and others) have been at the forefront, warning of the dangers of dental materials including mercury. Despite the overwhelming evidence of the dangers of these materials, these doctors have been persecuted by the mainstream dental community for speaking out against toxic dental practices.

The American Dental Association has lost credibility with the public at this point because it refuses to admit that amalgams are toxic and dangerous. The State of California for example, has deemed that the levels of mercury should be ten times lower than the current recommendations of the EPA (Environmental Planning Agency).

The risk assessment by scientists estimates that 120 million Americans have exceeded the maximum safe dose of mercury. Assessment of toxic metal levels can be made by your doctor. These tests however, are not simple blood tests. They require a chelating agent be administered to pull the metals from the tissues and assessed from the urinary clearance. The mercury and other toxic metals (lead, cadmium and arsenic—the test measures 17 different kinds) can be chelated out with intravenous and oral chelation agents.

Oral spirochete infections and bacteria are implicated in heart disease, diabetes, as well as central nervous system diseases. These bugs secrete small molecules that enhance inflammation and cause autoimmune disease. It is estimated that there are over 105 disease conditions associated with autoimmune disorders.

There have been more than fifty species of spirochetes identified in the oral cavity alone. Clostridium difficile, mycoplasma, human papilloma virus and other pathogens may cause disease as they also colonize in the mouth. Many of these have been implicated as a cause of Alzheimer's disease. There are laboratories that specialize in diagnosing bacterial burdens in the mouth, and identifying the exact species.

As a causal etiology, infection is one that is most intriguing to me as this paradigm fits the medical model best. Yet there is very little research in the area of infectious diseases as a cause of Alzheimer's disease. There have been viruses; mycoplasma and chlamydia implicated in both ALS and Alzheimer's disease, but spirochetes (bacteria known to be pathogens) seem to show the most promising cause and effect relationship.

The old hallmark disease of syphilis, which is caused by spirochetes, is a similar pathology to Alzheimer's disease, and has the tangles and plaque as part and parcel of the disease. We have known of this relationship for years and hence we encourage doctors to medicate patients with this disease early and until it is totally eradicated. We know if the condition turns into tertiary (chronic) syphilis, paralysis and dementia will follow.

Lyme's disease is also caused from spirochetes and renders a similar pathology. The incidence of tick bites has increased dramatically in recent years. Lyme's disease has contributed a lot of controversy in the medical community as to what is the best diagnostic test, what medications are most effective, length of treatment, when should treatment stop, when can a cure be assured, etc. Unlike syphilis, there has been no agreement as to treatment duration and measuring success through laboratory testing for Lyme's disease.

We do not know how many patients have not been treated properly, or never knew if they had Lyme's disease. They never developed a rash or target lesion. They may have only had prolonged flu like symptoms but went on to develop Alzheimer's disease or ALS.

In a scientific review of 495 patients with Alzheimer's disease, 451 of these patients (91.1%) of the samples were positive for spirochetes. In one study of 16 patients with Alzheimer's disease, 14 of 16 showed periodontal (oral) spirochetes. In many of these cases there were more than one species of spirochetes present capable of causing the classical pathology of Alzheimer's disease.

Spirochetes may access the brain through the nose and upper sinuses. The **cribriform plate** of the ethmoid bone, a small bone that forms part of the eye sockets and the nasal cavity, has small holes in it through which the periodontal spirochetes can pass into the forebrain. It is unfortunate that dentists do not preach to their patients that spirochetes, bacteria, and other bugs are the cause of systemic disease.

Diabetes, obesity, and cardiovascular disease are all associated with oral spirochetes. Dentists seem to concentrate on plaque caused from smoking or too much coffee as the cause of the biofilm and plaque turning into gingivitis, bone and tooth loss, and dental cavities. The real cause of this biofilm is bacteria, which multiplies in the pockets between the teeth and the gums where they do indeed cause disease. If my patients have gum disease, I know they may also have cardiovascular disease.

It may just be the spirochete disease we associate with Alzheimer's is really a sister infection from the mouth.

Action Plan:
If you have a "drill and fill" dentist, find a new one that is interested in prevention of disease. Get your mouth cleaned up, get rid of amalgam fillings, root canal teeth and any crowns that have an amalgam underlining. A good dentist is difficult to find, but they are available with a little research.

Not long ago, I had a slight discoloring of my gum. I thought I had replaced all of the amalgam fillings years ago and gotten all of the metal out of my mouth. Much to my surprise, I had a crown that had an underlining of amalgam. It taught me that I really need to question what was going into my mouth.

47

There is a special technique used to get amalgams out of your mouth. Verify that your dentist is familiar with this technique, as the drilling done in the amalgam removal will aerosolize the mercury, and when inhaled, can really make you sick.

Incidentally, the old filling materials are treated and disposed of as dangerous toxic waste.

I treat these conditions by using a laser to remove the plaque (biofilm) on the teeth, which limits the pockets where the spirochetes and other bacteria multiply. Use a mouth wash twice per day that will kill the bugs in the mouth. There are several good Tea Tree oil mouth washes available over the internet or in your health food store. This will address the biofilm and limit replication of bugs in the mouth.

The most effective way to kill the bacteria, including spirochetes, is to use a combination of 3% hydrogen peroxide and baking soda. Dip your brush in the peroxide first then into the baking soda, which will stick to the brush; brush, swish, and rinse. It sounds a little strange at first, as we are used to the sweet fluoride tasting toothpaste. You will eventually find it to be refreshing, as it cleans your teeth and kills the bugs in your mouth.

In addition to practicing good dental hygiene, I use a kefir drink daily which is loaded with good bacteria to wash my vitamins down. Make sure you buy organic, non-pasteurized (raw milk if possible) kefir, and do not use the nonfat/low fat products that are sold as these are likely hydrogenated and hence toxic to the body.

In chronic Lyme disease it is my opinion that unless there are symptoms of current infection like fever and flu-like symptoms it is better to enhance the patient's own immune system and avoid using long term antibiotics therapies. Having said this, recent research finds, ceftriaxone, an antibiotic used to treat Lyme disease was found to remove plaques from the brain. This would seem to indicate that a test for Lyme disease is mandatory in any case of dementia. To treat chronic Lyme disease look at the "Buhner Protocol". There are several web sites for information on this protocol on the internet.

—NOTES—

Tangles and Plaque

The pathological signs and symptoms of progressive brain atrophy, dementia, physical and cognitive dysfunction, and tangles and plaques in the brain, are very likely epigenetic (environmental).

I believe the scientific community has established that there is more than one factor that causes Alzheimer's disease.

There are a small number of cases associated with genetic abnormalities and the **apolipoprotein** (ApoE4). If a person has this inherited risk factor, they have an increased chance of acquiring Alzheimer's disease. Your doctor can check for ApoE4 and perform gene testing to see if you are predisposed to Alzheimer's disease.

But I also believe tangles and plaque contribute greatly to the inability of the neurological structures to keep up with the repair process of neurological tissue. Tangles and plaque come from either generating too much debris or failure to remove the debris in a timely manner. Possible mitochondrial dysfunction (process of converting food energy into cell energy), enzyme deficiency, fatty acid problem, vitamin and mineral deficiency, vascular insufficiency and of course infections are all possible etiologies.

Amyloid plaque may also come from the liver. It is documented that the liver produces amyloid which can cross the blood brain barrier into the brain to create sticky plaque also. It no doubt has a relationship to type II diabetes and the liver pathology that exists in the liver of diabetics. This is why, at present, we call Alzheimer's disease type III diabetes, and why this metabolic problem needs to be addressed.

Along this same line is the repair of the myelin sheath (the major problem in multiple sclerosis). The myelin sheath is a fatty coating surrounding the axon of nerve cells helping the nerve to transmit impulses very rapidly. One analogy is to liken it to a fiber optic cable, able to transmit millions of impulses. Myelin is repaired and replaced on a regular basis and I believe this process is interrupted and dysfunctional because we do not consume the proper amount and type of fat in our diet. EPA and DHA, found in fish oils, are mandatory to supplement. Alzheimer's patients lack the nutrients mentioned above which are necessary for the successful repair process.

Much of the volume shrinkage in the brain we see on CAT scans is the loss of myelin on the neurons. The gray matter of the cerebrum has a lot of myelin as well as the myelin sheath surrounding tracts of the spinal cord. Without this fatty myelin sheath we cannot enjoy proper neurological function. This functional process is rerouted and the neurons slow neurological transmission. This accounts for the gradual slowing of the mental process, poor memory, and associated physical impairment as we age.

Oligodendrocytes are the nerve cells that make myelin and they contain much more iron than other nerve cells. When these cells do not function properly and undergo premature apoptosis (death), they release iron into the brain. Free iron in the brain is very toxic and this creates an environment full of free radicals which creates a vicious cycle of cell death. Although after age 40 we do not create new **myelin**, we do have an active repair process for the existing myelin.

There are schools of science that propose the problem in all chronic neurological disease is the regeneration, repair and removal of myelin byproducts. This is explained simply here but some scientists have good arguments for the "myelin theory" as a unifying principal for chronic neurological dysfunction due to:

- Neurotoxins
- Spirochetes
- Heavy metals
- Aerosols
- Haloids
- Drugs
- Anything that causes inflammation, cell death and dysfunction

The defense mechanisms of the body remove dead and dying cells and other cellular debris. Now the problem exists that after age thirty, we produce only sufficient stem cells to repair small wear and tear problems, and to establish new memory patterns. Our bodies do not manufacture enough stem cells to repair large damage as occurs in Alzheimer's and stroke.

Oftentimes, the cellular structures are not dead. They are merely nonfunctional and not transmitting neurological impulse as they should. This is when stem cells, if administered in sufficient quantities, can reprogram these nonfunctional cells and initiate the regeneration process.

Action Plan:

It is most important to clean up the underlying terrain by removing the causal etiologies.

Address your metabolic syndrome and diabetes as much of this amyloid plaque may be originating in the liver of type II diabetics. This is therapy we have today and with proper nutrition we may well be able to reverse some of the damage or at least halt the progression of all forms of dementia.

- Use NutraGen™ products (refer to Products Chapter) formulated to control the inflammation and supply the body with the nutrients to heal itself.

- Initiate a weight loss program that includes a 3-4 day fast to reset the immune system and some intermittent fasting will quickly provide weight loss results. If obesity is severe, a doctor supervised "human chorionic gonadotropin hormone diet" can be instituted. This is a doctor supervised diet that produces fat loss and can shed pounds in a very controlled manner.

- Eat a paleo type diet. Along with a paleo type diet, you will get the type II diabetes under control.

- Ensure you get enough fats, vitamins, minerals and proteins so there is sufficient nutrition to remove the plaque and repair the brain tissue.

- Control the inflammation in the body. The herbal formulas and pure omegas are proven to help control the inflammation in your brain.

The supplements formulated byNutraGen™ for this process will provide the necessary nutrients to help the body rebalance neurological tissue.

As mentioned earlier, there are several antibody drugs coming out which are aimed at removing amyloid plaque. These are the monotherapy approach I have talked about which we pray will work. The big "but" is if the amyloid is removed will cognitive function improve. Do not wait around for these drugs—get proactive and begin suggestions given in this book immediately.

—NOTES—

PART FOUR

Resolution – The Good News

Diet for Alzheimer's

Diets higher in fat and proteins are far more supportive at preserving brain function. Diets that are high in carbohydrates and sugars, place a person at greater risk for Alzheimer's disease.

A diet high in simple carbohydrates and sugars no doubt has to do with the high blood sugar levels found in patients suffering type II diabetes. This is why we call Alzheimer's disease type III diabetes.

There is an interesting caveat here. We have been encouraged to eat foods in the USDA food pyramid. A diet plan that promotes a high carbohydrate, low fat diet, both which appear to be contraindicated in order to maintain brain health. There is an excellent book that outlines the historical bad dietary advice we have received from our medical leaders over the last 50 years. A book called *The Big Fat Surprise* by Nina Teicholz, gives a detailed, well documented account of the dietary farce surrounding the cholesterol scare and the food pyramid debacle in the United States.

The recommended low fat diet over the past 50 years provided too little saturated fat and too little fish oil essential type fat (EPA and DHA) in our diets. DHA is the most prevalent fat in the brain, comprising over 40% of the fat in the brain. If you drained the water out of the brain, it would comprise 40% fat.

If you do not provide the body with the exact type of fat it needs, it utilizes an alternative foreign source we call a "renegade fat" which does not perform the same efficient function in the neuronal tissue. It is little wonder that there are so many neurological diseases, as we have been consuming diets low in fat insufficient to rejuvenate and repair the neurons in the brain.

An olive oil derived phenolic component shows some promise as a neuro-protective factor for the neurons as it seems to delay neuron death. Fresh extra-virgin organic olive oil that has not turned rancid should be included in our diets. Organic coconut oil is a good saturated fat and should be included in the diet. Organic eggs are a great source of lecithin and fats, and should be included in the diet.

One should stay away from the vegetable oils like corn oil, safflower oil, soybean oil and other vegetable oils as these oils have proven to be a danger to our health, and have been our undoing. They have been unwisely placed into our food and have replaced the necessary saturated fats to build healthy bodies.

Eat good quality protein from grass-fed, hormone-free beef, bison or wild game: deer, elk and pheasant. If you eat chicken make sure it is free range chicken grown without antibiotics and hormones, and organically fed. Eat deep water fish or wild caught salmon and trout. Farm raised fish are inoculated with chemicals to keep the disease under control and not have them die while in captivity.

Action Plan:
There are several new books written recently on the benefits of the "Paleolithic diet," essentially a caveman-type diet — low in carbs and grains and higher in fat (40%), and proteins (30%) as a

daily food source. See appendix as there are slight differences in the books, but the same basic principles apply.

Totally avoid GMO (genetically modified foods) as I believe these cause cancer and dysregulation of the intestinal tract flora and immune system dysfunction. The NutraGen™ Pure Greens™, Pure Aomega Plus™, DHA/EPA Oil, and other products contained in the foundational status package are formulated to help support you with all the necessary nutrients required to make new neural tissue and to heal nonfunctional existing tissue.

In general, neurological diseases do better on a ketosis type diet. A good explanation of how it works can be found on the internet by searching "Ketogenic diet 101" where numerous websites can be found.

—NOTES—

Mitochondrial Dysfunction

Mitochondria are the power houses of a cell. They are organelles (little organs) within the cell that produce the body's energy.

When these organelles are stressed, due to excessive exposure to toxic drugs, aerosols, anesthetics, toxic metals, too much exercise and other substances mentioned in the previous discussion, the mitochondria get stressed and cannot function normally. It is due to this malfunction that they then produce free radicals. Free radicals are unpaired electrons which create havoc within the cell, producing amyloid, a substance that disrupts neuronal function and causes neuronal death.

Free radicals affect the ability of the cell to manufacture energy. This dysfunction also creates inflammation within the brain, which further advances neuronal death. The production of energy by the mitochondria is dependent on numerous vitamins and nutritional substances, like CoQ10, to produce energy for normal function.

Vitamins necessary for normal function are: B^1, B^2, B^3, B^6, B^{12} and folic acid. They are antioxidants and lower the neurotoxic byproducts like homocysteine, and lessen inflammation within the brain. B complex supplementation has shown to slow brain atrophy and lessen cognitive decline. It functions in a process called methylation, vital to neuron and DNA repair. Without methylation, one cannot repair the nervous system.

We must ensure that we provide the body with sufficient vitamin B complex vitamins, including nicotinamide, choline and inositol to guarantee the healing process can take place in the brain.

Action Plan:
Supplement with B complex vitamins. Since your doctor may not be schooled in nutrition I have identified an essential B complex formula for you. Even if you eat plenty of fresh vegetables, these vitamins are a special blend and vital to energy production and brain health.

Since B complex vitamins are water soluble, there is little possibility that one could overdose by taking too much of these vitamins. They will be eliminated in the urine if the body gets more than it can use.

Vitamin B^{12} and folic acid are another story, they can be measured in the blood and proper levels can be achieved either orally or by intramuscular injection. There are a high percentage of seniors (approximately 25%) that cannot convert the folic acid in their system and require a special formula called "five-methyl-tetra-hydro-folate." It is a mouthful and will be abbreviated on the supplement bottle in the health food store as 5MTHF. B^{12} and folic acid are important to the methylation process. NutraGen™ has included these in their products.

If the process does not function properly, the cell cannot make DNA or RNA proteins necessary for function and survival of the cell. Antioxidants too, are important as quenchers of free radicals within the cell. Some act in the fat soluble environment and some are water soluble. The brain needs both.

Neural Regeneration and Repair

Frequently in neurological diseases, the cells are not dead, they are just damaged and not functioning properly.

When I went to medical school, we were taught that adult **neurogenesis** (regeneration) was not possible. We use to recognize that children before age 6 could regain some brain function after a head injury but as adults there was no hope for neurological recovery.

With the advent of stem cell research in the past decade, we have discovered the brain can recover by making a small number of stem cells to be used for maintenance of neurological structures and establishing new memory circuits. However, if there is a great deal of damage, like in a stroke, these few stem cells are simply not sufficient to rejuvenate a large area of damage to the neurological tissue.

When I administer a large dose of neural stem cells to brain injury patients, the neurological tissue which is living but not functioning properly gets reprogrammed by the new stem cells and begins to function again. The administered stem cells secrete small signaling molecules which help to jump start the neural healing process. There is proof that these cells actually engraft and secrete the appropriate neurotransmitter substances.

With the administration of stem cells for neurological conditions, especially:

- stroke

- traumatic brain injury (TBI)

- spinal cord injury

we are able to rewrite the book on how these neurological conditions can heal. Because these are more of an acute injury, with a known etiology, they respond differently than do chronic disease processes.

The chronic disease conditions may have no known etiology or have multiple etiologies, and the underlying terrain of the patient's health is not stable. Cleaning up the patient's ongoing toxic environment may well be a prerequisite before response can be measured. Ongoing problems like:

- spirochete infection

- heavy metal toxicity

- dietary deficiencies

- exposures to aerosols

- other environmental toxins

These problems may need to be addressed before we can optimize the response to therapy.

Future stem cell research on humans will determine what type of stem cells will be used, how many of each cell will be required for a treatment, how often they should be administered, and when treatment is optimized.

I believe with the correct formula of stem cells, physical therapy, medications, nutritional supplementations, and metabolic support, we can rehabilitate and make a dramatic change in the cognitive and functional recovery of patients with Alzheimer's disease not experienced before in neurology.

Action Plan:
There is hope. Follow a plan to clean up the terrain of the body.

- Institute proper nutrition, avoid exposure to toxic substances, and avoid unnecessary drugs, anesthetics and aerosols.

- Make every attempt to rid the body of toxic metals and ensure that you clean the bacteria and remove the metals from your mouth.

- Get tested for heavy metals load (lead, mercury, and other toxic metals) in your body. If the levels are high rid the body of these toxic metals via intravenous chelation or certainly an oral chelation substance.

- Begin on the nutritional substances NutraGen™ formulated for this purpose to help the body detoxify and provide the body with the healing substances it needs.

- It is a good idea to investigate stem cell therapy to repair and regenerate the damaged brain. There are many clinical trials ongoing here in the United States and throughout the world.

I believe the USFDA will fast track stem cell administration for many "no option" medical conditions. Remember you need the correct type of stem cells. One size does not fit all. You may need a nerve stem cell, vascular bone marrow stem cell, a muscle stem cell, or other specific stem cell to treat your condition.

Use the NutraGen™ Pure Greens™ and Pure Digestion™ to liver detoxification and balance intestinal function. Use essential oils and B complexes that will allow the body to repair itself. Remember the micro environment in the gut reflects brain function. Ensure you treat the gut pathology so that the brain can heal itself. Get a comprehensive stool analysis, balance the flora in the gut which will decrease systemic and brain inflammation.

Antioxidants

It is important to note, the generation of free radical "oxidation" is a normal function of all cells. The body needs some free radicals as they are normal initiators of the metabolic process.

It is when one generates too many free radicals, the body experiences "oxidative stress." Oxidative stress can be:

- Physical stress as in too many marathons

- Drug stress as in too many medications

- Street drugs or alcohol abuse

- Dietary imbalances resulting in ongoing pathology in the cell which can lead to cell death

- Exposure to cigarette smoke

- Infections of all types

I mentioned earlier "oxidative stress" is a major cause of free radicals formation and neuronal death. This may be due to a compensatory system that is overloaded, faulty metabolism due to mitochondrial malfunction or a shortage of anti-oxidant vitamins, like vitamin C and vitamin E (which is the major fat soluble vitamin). Anti-oxidants are critical to quenching the damaging free radicals which are generated by neuronal cell stress.

Science has discovered new sources of anti-oxidants that we refer to as **phytonutrients**. These are frequently found in fruits and vegetables, and can be extracted, concentrated, and placed into our food as supplements. They have qualities that are desirable as quenchers of free radicals, which assist the body in healing and maintenance of optimal function.

These phytonutrients are frequently contained in green drinks. The content of these drinks, the source organic vs genetically modified food, as well as the extraction method, are all important to make them as effective as possible and ensure that they not do more harm than good. There has been research that finds that they can help:

- Modulate blood sugar in type II diabetes

- Quench the viruses in hepatitis C

- Assist the endothelium in vascular disease

- Lower blood pressure

And many more claims. In order to make a claim that a phytonutrient is effective in a certain condition, one must provide the FDA with research that proves the claim.

Action Plan:
Because there are hundreds of phytonutrient, it is confusing to most people as to what they should take. To simplify the problem NutraGen™ had a Pure Greens™ product made with the best ingredients that will achieve optimal results. In order to avoid conflict with the FDA regulatory bodies, NutraGen™ makes the following statement: "phytonutrients may assist the body in maintaining a healthy nervous system."

I do know that many phytonutrients are the medicines of the future. They will be used to control blood sugar, inflammation, and neurological conditions. Some ginsenosides from Ginseng for example, have proven to be effective as neuroregenerative and neuroprotective phytonutrients.

The general statement that the phytonutrient may have a *beneficial effect* on certain conditions without actually making a claim for a disease relationship satisfies the FDA.

Some of these nutrients no doubt, will turn into the drugs of the future. Healthy mitochondrial function depends on:

- CoQ10

- Vitamins

- Certain amino acids (proteins)

- Minerals like magnesium, chromium, selenium and zinc

The cornerstone of healthy neurological function, these phytonutrients are contained in the NutraGen™ Pure Greens™ product. See product description in the back of the book.

—NOTES—

Inflammation

Quelling inflammation is necessary to prevent neural destruction by an over-active immune system and provide an environment conducive to the healing process.

There have been studies suggesting that aspirin and other nonsteroidal anti-inflammatories (NSAID) such as Ibuprofen and Naproxen, are effective to lower inflammation and prolong neuron life. The problem is these drugs have side effects such as bleeding and gastro-intestinal inflammation, causing over 16,000 deaths in the US annually.

There are tens of thousands of hospitalizations and deaths in the US yearly as a result of NSAID use. Certain herbs like curcumin have proven to have great anti-inflammatory benefits and are virtually free of side effects. Having said this, one should adhere to the instructions on the bottle and if you are combining these, by using more than one herb at a time, consult a health care practitioner. Combining certain medications and herbs may be contradictive. Again, consult with a health care practitioner who has knowledge in this area.

If a product is making claims they work as an anti-inflammatory agent, the manufacturer has to prove it, using research that will satisfy the FDA. I also use enzymes as anti-inflammatory agents in the intestines like pancreatin, betaine, pepsin, bromelain and ox bile. The enzymes, if taken in high enough dosages, are effective to lower inflammation in the intestine where most of the immune system is located.

It is thought some herbs have the ability to dissolve the amyloid plaque as they are proven to cross the blood brain barrier to have a profound anti-inflammatory effect. Herbs like turmeric, boswellia and ginger (as used in NutraGen™ Pure InflaMedix™ product) have a systemic effect. In my opinion these can replace aspirin and NSAID drugs.

One can see that a comprehensive approach to Alzheimer's disease treatment is required and can be done naturally. The natural approach however must attempt to address and treat as many of the underlying factors as possible. Because there are multiple causal etiologies for inflammation and the biochemical and structural changes that are occurring in the brain, we need to use multiple supplements to address the problems.

We know that if we use anti-inflammatory medications, we can salvage neurons and delay cell death. I discussed earlier that infections (spirochetes infection) cause inflammation. Reactive oxygen species (a byproduct of the body's own oxygen metabolism) cause inflammation and neuron death from toxic metals like mercury, haloids, aluminum and fluoride—really any environmental stresses. All these work to cause inflammation in the brain and early neuronal cell death. With inflammation, there is activation of the immune system cells in the brain. These brain cells are called microglia.

The microglia becomes activated by dead and dying cells, as well as the foreign substances in the brain like toxic metals and infectious agents. Their activation results in a vicious cycle as they secrete inflammatory signaling molecules to create more inflammation. Over a period of months to years, a vicious cycle

74

occurs and a patient loses many millions of viable neurons. Since there are millions of neurons in the brain, there can be a loss of millions before a there is a notable clinical neurological deficit which can be recognized by the patient's family members.

Action Plan:

It is essential to clean up the underlying bodily terrain by eliminating bacteria, toxic metals, haloids and supplying the body with proper phytonutrients, vitamins and minerals required for efficient mitochondrial function. We expect when we eliminate the etiologies that cause neurological death this will create an environment for healing to take place and for the brain tissue to be reprogrammed by stem cell transplantation.

NutraGen™ has created a herbal product that addresses inflammation, Pure InflaMedix™, and of the opinion it is as effective as non-steroidal anti-inflammatory medications without unwanted side effects.

Begin with the NutraGen™ foundation products such as Pure Cleanse Plus™ to help support liver detoxification and Pure Digestion Plus™ for intestinal support. This will help to negate systemic inflammation and normalize bowel function. Remember that most of the immune system is contained in the intestines. It is necessary to control bowel function to achieve overall health.

—NOTES—

Endothelial Dysfunction

Endothelial dysfunction does not occur in a vacuum. If one organ is symptomatic, like your heart, there is a problem throughout the whole body.

In our previous discussion, we suggested there is a definite vascular component to Alzheimer's disease. The endothelium is a singular layer of cells inside your arteries which acts as the largest hormone secretor in the body.

Science has found that the endothelial layer secretes multiple signaling molecules which have an enormous impact on body function. If you have a plugged up artery in your heart or possibly have a stent in your heart, you have a systemic vascular problem that should be addressed immediately.

The problem starts with this inner lining of the artery, but eventually this inflammation blocks the whole of the artery (small ones get plugged first). You do not have to wait until you have a problem. You can ask your doctor to do the tests that will give you an assessment of your endothelial health. If he/she does not know what you are talking about, find a doctor who does and will help you.

The three assessments are:

- Blood tests to measure inflammation, and small molecule products that have to do with the condition of the arteries. (See Singulex Labs at www.singulex.com).

- Ultra sound test for carotid intimal thickness (carotids are the neck arteries) which is a very accurate measurement of the arterial intimal thickness and calcification.

- Noninvasive testing, pulsed wave analysis

Remember, if these are abnormal, then there are problems with your whole arterial system.

On a daily basis, cardiologists place stents in the heart arteries and routinely prescribe statin drugs which are supposed to help the endothelium. This however presents a new problem as statins cause dementia and eye disease. In my opinion, this is a bad tradeoff, especially when there are more effective treatments available. More effective and simple solutions then statin drugs are:

- Removing toxic metals from the blood
- Controlling your metabolic syndrome/diabetes
- Adding anti-oxidants to your diet
- Taking supplements that boost nitric oxide
- Stop smoking

Endothelial dysfunction starts in the blood vessels (endothelium) causing narrowing of the blood vessels (arteriosclerosis). It is this compromise in blood flow that causes vascular dementia. The endothelium when inflamed secretes numerous inflammatory cytokines and proteins causing systemic inflammation.

Type II diabetes and obesity also cause endothelial inflammation as excess fat secretes inflammatory molecules. All type II diabetics and obese patients have endothelial dysfunction and have systemic inflammation which leads to dementia.

Action Plan:
The solution is to get the type II diabetes under control. If you are a smoker, stop. If your blood pressure is high have your doctor prescribe an ACE inhibitor medication to get it under control. Acheive optimal weight by beginning a paleo type diet, get regular exercise and decrease stress.

Have your doctor order an endothelial blood panel. Singulex labs has a very good one. You can look these tests up at www.Singulex.com, under endothelial dysfunction. There are some general tests like hsCRP and homocysteine that also are markers for endothelial inflammation. These tests are a great way to get a baseline to measure future progress against.

Of course there are the high tech imaging devices like ultra sound, pet scans, CAT scans and MRI which combined with contrast medium (dye) that can image the vascular systems. Some clinics use a machine that uses a blood pressure cuff which inflates and deflates and the machine can interpret the flexibility of the vascular system. See Vendy's or Endopat machines for endothelial testing. This is a completely noninvasive way to test the vascular system.

Please see the diabetes plan at the end of this book and tests required to diagnose this disease, as endothelial dysfunction is the initiating process involved in hypertension and diabetes.

It is very important to address this issue as it is an underlying problem in systemic inflammation. Vascular dementia may be the cause of or a contributing factor to the dementia that you or your loved one is suffering from.

Address the inflammation in the vascular bed so that healing can begin. In addition to the above suggestions the NutraGen™ Pure Greens™ product and Pure InflaMedix™ anti-inflammatory herbal product are definitely indicated.

Nitric oxide has been a long overlooked supplement. It is commonly known that the amino acid arginine is converted by the body into nitric oxide. This conversion slows dramatically as we mature and in order to get enough, we must use a nitric oxide supplement. Because nitric oxide has such a profound effect on the endothelium (the lining of the blood vessels) it increases the circulation and thus has healing effects on many body systems. The NutraGen™ nutritional supplements specifically address this issue and are designed to help heal the endothelium.

Nitric oxide is the number one anti-oxidant in the vascular system. When we have sufficient amounts in the blood it has a profound effect on increasing circulation and thus has a healing effect on many body systems.

To get started healing the endothelium, please begin the NutraGen™ foundation products of Pure Greens™ and Pure Inflamex™ without delay. This new product derived from beet-root power and L-Citrulline can increase nitric oxide in the vascular bed and is worth taking.

Intestinal Flora

Most people think of the gut as a sewage disposal system, not as a living source of energy for the body. Also sixty percent of our immune system is contained in the gut.

I was going to begin this section by calling it "bugs in the gut," but for some reason people are uncomfortable with this subject. Thinking of billions of bacteria crawling around inside of our intestines is not a pleasant subject for most people.

Bacteria in your gut, however, have a big role in our overall health. They manufacture B complex vitamins, vitamin K, and medium short chained fats we use for energy. They convert waste food products into nutrients necessary for the body to function properly. So what is the problem?

- GMO foods
- Pesticides
- BPA plastics
- Synthetic food products
- Artificial sweeteners
- High carbohydrate diets
- Low fiber diets
- Infectious agents like bacteria, fungus and mycoplasma

- Deficient intake of beneficial flora and fiber

- Antibiotics

- Stomach medications

Processed foods also contain little fiber so critical to the functioning of the good bacteria in your gut. The essential flora has a direct impact on the production of many types of immune system cells.

Because we eat in restaurants, we are exposed to infectious diseases. Experts believe only 5% of food poisoning contracted in restaurants is reported with meat being highly suspect as it is:

- handled by numerous people,

- raised in unsanitary feed lots,

- fed synthetic foods laced with antibiotics.

This imbalance in flora (bad bacteria) creates inflammation in the intestines and causes numerous autoimmune diseases. Because most of the food we eat is highly processed, it lacks essential nutrients contained in raw unprocessed food. Of interest, most people get 90 percent of their nutrition from just 17 different food sources. Unless one is very careful of what they eat, most of the diets in the United States are deficient of good bacteria content and nutritional quality.

Our whole nation is advised to eat according to the food pyramid which has grains as the base of the pyramid and contains 70% carbohydrates, much of which are refined starches loaded with calories but devoid of significant nutrition. Processed foods also contain little fiber so critical to the functioning of the good bacteria in your gut.

There is a combination of elements that have caused a new wave of autoimmune diseases and hypersensitivity in the gut. These include:

- high-tech engineering of our food sources by creating genetically modified foods (GMO),

- undue emphasis on high carbohydrate grain-filled diets,

- altered content of grains, high in gluten and residual weed killer genetics from the seed,

- haptens generated by antibiotics fed to the animals and to humans, plastics, synthetic drugs, pathogenic bacteria in the gut, hormones fed to animals and toxic chemicals.

A recent research article claimed that certain abnormal bacterium was closely associated with coronary artery disease. Also noted recently is artificial sweeteners promoting abnormal pathogenic bacteria in the gut and limiting the growth of beneficial bacteria. Just when we thought we were limiting calories and eating healthy, we find these artificial sweeteners (Splenda, Equal, Sweet'NLow etc.) are contributing to our ill health.

Is gut bacteria important? Yes, your health depends on healthy gut function.

Action Plan:
First, get a comprehensive stool analysis to determine the gut flora balance and identify any pathogenic "disease-causing" bacteria. Your doctor can help you rid the gut of pathological bacteria and fungus, and balance the flora. Get on a high fiber diet and supplement some good fiber into your diet. Eat organic meats, fruits and vegetables.

Read labels and stay away from all GMO and synthetic hormone treated foods. I use good organic yogurt, kefir, and a product called Bio-K, available at the health food store.

Beware! Most "so-called" low fat yogurt is harmful to your body. It has all the natural good fat removed and sugar added. It is synthetic and made with hydrogenated milk with BFT growth hormone added to the cow's feed to force their system to produce more milk.

It is easy to make your own yogurt – use raw milk (or goat milk as it is hypoallergenic) and the Bio-K product mentioned above, and simple let it ferment for a day or two. This is so important NutraGen™ developed a special intestinal formula Pure Digestion Plus™ to support intestinal health. There are many internet sites for instructions and recipes so you can do your own yogurt.

Finally, totally eliminate artificial sweeteners from your diet.

Environment – Electro Magnetic Field

When I was born 70 years ago, there were approximately 1 billion people in the world. Now there are 7.3 billion and growing.

It is estimated that the world is sustainable with 9 billion people. Even today, we have much of Africa malnourished and much of Central and South America impoverished. The world has become an urbanized place where most of us live in or near a large city.

With this growth process, we have given up growing our own individual food supply and rely on others from all over the world to grow specific crops for us. Thus, we have no control over:

- Pesticides
- Fertilizers
- Storage and ripening techniques
- Which foods are GMO and which are not.
- Which foods are grown in toxic soil and are contaminated even before harvesting.

Food is handled multiple times before it gets to our plate, thereby increasing the probability of spreading infectious diseases.

Governments in these urbanized countries supply the populous with electricity, potable water, garbage and sewage disposal. This has lessened the plagues throughout the world, but has presented itself with an entirely different set of problems, unimagined in my youth.

Chlorine is in our water to kill the bacteria and make it drinkable from the tap. Fluoride is in the water because it supposedly prevents tooth decay and because it is financially profitable for certain companies. Both chlorine and fluoride are used, despite the fact both are toxic to our bodies and contribute to neurodegenerative diseases. There are alternative technologies to treat our water without chlorine and fluoride as these two halogens definitely promote neuro degeneration.

Electrical fields are an unprecedented new problem with the invention of high voltage electrical power lines and transformers strung out over the entire country. Microwave towers and highline wires transmit a variety of high frequency currents all of which have a detrimental impact on our bodies. It is virtually impossible to find an organic space without them. Add to this:

- Electrical appliances (microwave ovens)
- Air conditioners
- Computers in automobiles
- Computers in the office and home
- Televisions, cell phones and cell towers
- Wi-Fi currents everywhere we go

All emitting electrical frequencies, which are foreign to and detrimental to the body.

The full extent of this frequency disruption is unknown or at the very least, we are in denial of their possible impact. The use of cell phones in Sweden and Norway are limited in children under 18 years of age. This gives you some idea of how some of the educated world thinks of current emitted from cell phones.

It is important to note the body is electric. Our cells operate using electrical charges. Proteins, minerals, electrolytes like sodium and potassium all have small electrical charges. The problem is too little recharging of the body systems with low voltage like that given off by the earth. Too much electrical charging of higher voltage like cell phone towers, Wi-Fi fields, and high voltage wires can dramatically affect the way the body functions.

Action Plan:
Although we cannot escape all of these frequencies, we can limit our time in front of the computer and television, and eliminate frequencies while we sleep.

We can ensure there are no electrical devices in the bedroom – no televisions, computers, air conditioners, cell phones etc. to interrupt our sleep patterns. Talk on cell phones only when necessary, use the speaker option and do not carry them in close proximity to your body.

Pulsed electrical magnetic frequency (PEMF) devices are recommended for all neurological conditions. See www.DrPawluk.com for more information. This battery-operated device reconnects your body with the frequencies of the earth. Under normal circumstances, if we go barefoot with our feet on the earth, this would automatically happen.

Our lifestyle of constantly wearing shoes and constantly walking on solid surfaces does not lend itself to this natural connection to the ground. A PEMF device (low magnetic field) will reconnect you with mother earth and help to heal neuro-degenerative diseases. I recommend these devices in all neuro-degenerative diseases.

Sleep

Sleep is an often overlooked cause of neurological function. If you are sleep deprived your brain cannot function properly.

There is an on/off switching process in the brain. During the daytime, a serotonin/dopamine switch is turned-on. In the evening, this switch is turned-off while the growth hormone melatonin, and other brain derived growth factors are secreted into the general circulation. These hormones are powerful and necessary for the body to function properly.

Come daytime again this switching process is reversed whereby the growth hormone, melatonin, and other growth factors are turned-off, and the serotonin/dopamine are once again turned-on. In this way the body can rebalance itself.

If a person does not get sufficient sleep it affects this on/off switching. Both the daytime, and the nighttime hormones are interrupted and the body cannot function properly.

If there is inflammation in the body, it drives the cortisol levels up. Cortisol is the stress hormone when elevated can destroy memory and nerve tissue. This sleep period if interrupted does not allow the brain to lay down new memory and hormones to re-balance themselves.

By controlling stress and inflammation, patients can get a much better night's sleep.

Most scientists believe that eight hours sleep is required to rebalance hormones allowing for the memories to be programmed into the brain. Patients who sleep better have performed better on memory tests than people who sleep poorly.

Action Plan:
Simply go to bed earlier. Early enough that when morning comes you do not require an alarm clock to wake up. You wake up on your own at a time well ahead of what is required for you to start your day. This routine is much less stressful and you will now know your individual biological clock setting.

Avoid too much stimulation prior to bed such as TV. Go to website www.bettersleep.com for many helpful tips for better sleep.

For further help, consult with a pulmonary specialist who may do a sleep study in a laboratory or at home. You may have sleep apnea and require what is known as a continuous positive airway pressure (CPAP) machine. Natural herbal supplements such as melatonin may be enough. Again do your research and consult an herbalist or alternative medicine practitioner.

Social Interaction, Mind Stimulation and Exercise

Keeping the mind active also appears to be important to maintain and re-establish the neuronal connections.

It is important to get sufficient aerobic exercise. Physical exercise has been found to enhance cognitive function. It helps the circulation especially in the back part of the brain and can help memory. Exercising the mind with decision-making games, exercises the front of the brain and helps with executive function and decision making.

Exercise also prevents muscle loss and thus prevents frailty, a major causes of death in the elderly. Exercise enhances circulation and the release of certain endorphins critical to brain stimulation.

In addition to helping to maintain weight, there are a lot of secondary effects obtained by exercise. Growth factors, cytokines, and hormones are enhanced in patients who get regular aerobic exercise.

Action Plan:
Spend at least 30 minutes every other day in some form of aerobic exercise (walking, swimming, etc.)

There are a host of suggestions for keeping the mind active—crossword puzzles, card games, reading and learning new languages etc.

Social interaction with friends and family also seems to be important keeping elders an integral part of the social and family unit. There are several suggestions for ongoing social interaction which can be found on numerous Alzheimer's web sites www.alzheimer.org being one.

Medications worth Taking

"Prayer indeed is good, but while calling on the gods a man should himself lend a hand" — *Hippocrates.*

The following list of medications are worth taking.

Centrophenoxine:
This drug is used to treat senile dementia and Alzheimer's disease. It is an ester of dimethylethanolamine (DMAE) 4chlorphenoxyacetic acid (pCPA). DMAE is a natural substance found commonly in fish. pCPA is a synthetic compound and resembles a group of plant hormones called auxins. Interestingly, these plant hormones have growth factors that can affect the neurological tissues in a positive manner.

It is reported Centrophenoxine can actually dissolve the tangles and plaque found in Alzheimer's patients. It works as an antioxidant, keeping membranes fluid and also increases choline availability. This drug is a natural product (no synthetic component) that has a high level of safety and should be a primary drug on the list for treatment of Alzheimer's and other dementias.

In elderly patients Centrophenoxine has been shown to clinically improve memory. It also has been shown to improve the lipid (fat) content so important to the membrane of the neural cell. Have your doctor check it out on the internet as there are some cautions for patients with severe high blood pressure and patients suffering from epilepsy. I believe this is a drug worth a try.

Deprenyl:
Deprenyl is effective in Parkinson's disease and dementia. It has shown to be neuroprotective and a cognitive function enhancer in animal studies. There are very few contraindications to therapy. I have found that it seems to wake up the synaptic sites in the brain.

I have written many prescriptions for the drug Deprenyl. It has several commercial names – Selegiline, Emsan (transdermal patch), Rasagiline, Eldepryl and there are likely a few more. It is a dopamine agonist, which by definition is involved in any movements of the body. Deprenyl is a monoamine oxidase B and at higher doses, an A inhibitor.

Hydergine:
Hydergine has been used for years for dementia, or age-related cognitive dysfunction. It is derived from three sub-groups of ergoloid mesylate. This drug no doubt has an effect on the vasculature in Alzheimer's disease. As I stated earlier, at least 30% of dementias have a vascular component-vascular insufficiency or arteriosclerosis.

Memantine:
Memantine is marketed under the name Ebixia. The indications for this medication are for moderate Alzheimer's disease, but there are no claims for a cure with this drug. It has been claimed to control the amount of glutamate, a neurotransmitter which enhances the communication between the cells. Too much glutamate causes an irritation and inflammation of the neurons. Ebixia can improve memory and functioning. Clinical studies show improvements and slowing of the progression of

Alzheimer's disease. However, this medication does have some side effects your doctor should discuss with you.

Aricept:
Aricept (donepezil) is an acetylcholinesterase inhibitor intended for all stages of dementia and Alzheimer's disease. Acetylcholine is a neurotransmitter (substance that enhances the nerve transmission) between the nerve cells. In an earlier portion of the book we discussed choline, a member of the B vitamin family when taken orally, can enhance memory.

Choline:
Choline increases the duration of time that acetylcholine is available in the synapse (area between two nerve cells), thereby improving the functioning of patients with dementias. There are several drugs that are acetylcholinesterase inhibitors; a few are: Galantamine, Rivastigmine and Neostigmine. They all work in a similar manner, but they all have numerous side affects you need to discuss with your doctor. Whereby Choline is a naturally occurring vitamin without the side effects.

Metformin:
Metformin is FDA approved for type II diabetes. There have been numerous diabetes drugs pulled from the market or drug companies were forced to place a black box warning on their labels. Metformin however has been a recommended drug in my practice for some time. It has been considered as a "smart drug" (a drug that promotes brain health) by many anti-aging doctors.

As I mentioned in the diabetes chapter, Alzheimer's disease is referred to as type III diabetes. This is because the neurons and other cells in the brain depend on glucose as an energy source. In Alzheimer's disease, the brain cells develop insulin resistance. This means the brain cells resist the entry of glucose into the cell, much the same as in the periphery where the muscle cells (which burn most of the glucose in the body) develop insulin resistance. Insulin resistance is one of the first metabolic malfunctions of the muscle cells and likely coincides with the pathology of insulin resistance in the brain.

Metformin also controls blood sugar swings, helps with weight control, and lipid balance. A side effect of nausea and upset stomach is common at higher dosages.

Hormones:
I have previously mentioned the importance of hormones as they progressively decline in our bodies as we age. Hormones control the function of every organ system in the body. It may well be the progressive decline of hormones with age is precipitated by the slowdown in neuronal function as we age.

The feedback control mechanism that controls virtually all systemic hormones is located in the brain. Control of major hormones works like this: the brain secretes a releasing hormone that talks to the pituitary gland (master gland of the body) which then instructs an endocrine organ (like the thyroid, adrenal gland, ovary, etc.) to secrete the appropriate amount of hormone into the blood which allows for optimal function of the tissues governed by the organ. This is a very precise system that seems to fail as we age. We lose about 2-3% of this hormone secreting capacity per year from age thirty. So at age sixty one has lost at least one half of the hormones we possess at age thirty.

This chronic shortage of hormones is responsible for the general slowing of total body systems as we age. Many doctors believe that if we keep the major hormones in a good therapeutic range it will slow the aging process and help one to maintain good physical and cognitive function until we die. The chronic Hypothalamic

Pituitary Axis (HPA) is what we call the communication between the brain control centers and the pituitary gland. and are likely influenced by:

- Free radicals
- Insulin resistance in the brain cells
- Stress hormones like cortisol
- Lack of sleep and aerobic exercise

There does not seem to be any contraindications to keeping hormones in a good therapeutic range, with an exception to this statement as some doctors limit some hormones in cancer patients. Talk to a doctor about your health. One who is knowledgeable in the prescribing of natural bio-identical hormones.

As mentioned previously, I use a more natural approach in supplementing hormones to optimize function. Remember hormones are the control mechanisms for all vital organs. They control mood, libido, mental energy, memory, physical strength, cardiac muscle strength and endurance. Many schools of thought believe when we completely deplete our hormones, we die.

There are several hormones worth consideration and may need to be balanced like: growth hormone, melanocyte stimulating hormone, melatonin, DHEA, cortisol, estrogens, progesterone, testosterone, aldosterone, all need to be checked and balanced.

Get your hormones balanced and use bio-identical hormones, or use a full spectrum thyroid replacement drug like Amour's thyroid or Westroid as thyroid replacement verses a synthetic thyroid replacement. The sex hormones like estrogen, and testosterone are essential for optimal brain function while pregnenlone and progesterone are considered to be neurotransmitters in the brain. These are vital to survival and can be tested to place your body in the optimal range.

Special Vitamins:
I mention these special forms of vitamins under the drug section as we have very good scientific data that they are of utmost importance to the function of the nerve cell. There are other nutritionals that are important as well and they will be covered under the nutritional section of the book.

Niagen is a special form of niacin, a B complex vitamin. B complex vitamins play a vital role in the production of energy. The mitochondria use them in their energy cycle to produce ATP (adenosine triphosphate), the actual chemical substance that the body burns for fuel. Niacin, niacinamide and nicotinic acid are all forms of vitamin B3 used by the body, but research found that a specially prepared molecule called nicotinamide riboside is the most readily avalable form of niacin that can be immediately utilized by the mitochondria in the brain to produce energy.

Choline is a member of the B complex family and along with inositol is vital to good brain function. Choline is the principal component of acetylcholine, the primary neurotransmitter involved in Alzheimer's disease and the chemical that Alzheimer's medications are attempting to target. There are some herbs, like ginkgo biloba and ginseng that have proven to stimulate acetylcholine.

Benfotamine is another one of the B complex vitamins. It is a special form of thiamine (B1) which is fat soluble. Most of the B complex vitamins are water soluble and because of this, the amount that can be absorbed in the intestines is limited, only about 17% of the water soluble type gets absorbed. However, this is not a problem with the fat soluble form of thiamine, over 80% gets absorbed. Benefotamine has the unique ability to alleviate cerebral oxidative damage and buildup of cellular debris in the neurons of the brain. Look at www.benfotamine.com. There are hundreds of scientific articles utilizing this form of B1 for things like peripheral neuropathy (numbness in the hands and feet).

ACE and ARB are hypertension drugs. ACE (angiotensin converting enzymes) and ARB (angiotensin receptor blockers) are thought to be neuro protective and have a small effect on reducing cognitive decline. These hypertension drugs are important to blood pressure control and important in preventing stroke and further organ degeneration. Blood pressure control is an important part of the therapy in Alzheimer's disease. It seems that high blood pressure in midlife compounds the chances to develop Alzheimer's in later life. It was reported recently that a high protein diet decreased blood pressure, so ensure that you get enough high quality meat in your diet. NutraGen™, Pure Plant Protein™ is an excellent source of hypoallergenic protein. Cardiac function is directly linked to brain function. The better heart function the less likely one is to develop dementia.

Lithium has long been used for neurological disorders, but its exact mechanism of action is unknown. We use low dose therapy (thirty milligrams) so that the user does not have to have their lithium levels checked. It likely helps to repair and recycle neurons and optimize mitochondrial function.

Antibiotics may be helpful, especially those that can pass the blood brain barrier (minocycline). In some studies, antibiotics seemed to reduce cognitive decline in some patients. In this study the antibiotic therapy was of long term, one year duration. Recently an antibiotic called ceftriaxone was found to remove plaques from the brain. I use oxygen therapies; hydrogen peroxide and ozone IV (intravenous) as these cross the blood brain barrier and can kill viruses, bacteria and the most likely invading etiology, like spirochetes.

Insulin especially the nasal administered type, seems to be indicated especially where we have type II diabetes present. Since with Alzheimer's there is insulin resistance in the brain, there is clear indication that this makes good medical sense to use insulin, at the very least on a trial basis.

Stem cell factors BDNF (brain derived nerve factor), GDNF (Glial derived nerve factor), NGF (nerve growth factor), and FGF2 (fibroblast growth factor) are small molecules secreted by neural stem cells and have been isolated from the cultivation of nerve stem cells (neurons and glial stem cells). These factors have been found to be effective in stimulating nerve function. They have been patented and have not yet been approved for human use in the United States. They are worth mentioning here, as they are on the horizon and you should be aware of them. These would likely be administered as a nasal inhalant.

G-CSF (Granulocyte colony stimulating factor) is another small signaling molecule that has the ability to stimulate certain types of white blood cells. This likely works as the white blood cells fight infection and when activated, works much better than antibiotics as it activates the natural defense system of the body.

Nutrients worth Taking

Because pharmacological intervention has largely failed in its development of drugs to prevent, slow the progression of, or adequately treat Alzheimer's, there is now a call for lifestyle interventions.

In the year 2030, a hypertension drug company's prediction states 20% of the population in the US will be over age 65. It is well recognized there is a pressing need to find some answers to Alzheimer's dementia. Lifestyle interventions not only emphasize food and nutrition, diabetes control, exercise, weight loss and cognitive stimulation as a treatment but as a preventative intervention for dementia.

It is not surprising that we have gross nutritional deficiencies because Americans derive 80% of their nutrition from only seventeen foods. If one eliminates red meat or significantly reduces its intake, there will be a fat, protein, vitamin and mineral deficiency in the diet. Vegetarians on the other hand must be very cognitive of their food selection in order to get all the necessary nutrients for a balanced diet

It is interesting to note that many researchers are looking for the "missing link" to the mystery of Alzheimer's disease—that one missing molecule, if replaced, will make the cell run normally. The idea is, if a scientist can find the correct "key for the lock," they will find the answer. I believe, and I think you will agree, that we have identified numerous etiologies and that there could be multiple locks that will require different keys in order to regenerate cells so they will once again function normally.

In order to have compliance from my patients, I recommend NutraGen™ products including a Pure Greens™ product that incorporates many of the nutrients patients will be asked to take. This product will act to replace many of the nutritional deficiencies and provide the brain the proper nutrients to rejuvenate itself. There is also a NutraGen™ Pure Plant Protein™ product which can be mixed with the NutraGen™ Pure Greens™ or taken separately which will make compliance much easier and limit the number of separate pills that the patient must take to supply proper nutrition. The NutraGen™ Pure Aomega Plus™ is designed to give you the essential fats required to help the brain heal itself. Of course, one must include olive oil, coconut oil, and a variety of nuts. Saturated fats from meat are also required by all cells.

As I reviewed the research articles collected for this section of the book, I was amazed to find a plethora of information on each nutrient I'd planned to include. In the big overview of this research it is difficult to determine what the most important nutrient is. They all are linked together and are inter-dependent on each other. This combination is necessary to make the biochemistry of the cell work in an efficient fashion so the cells of the central nervous system (CNS) can perform its required genetic function.

To date, we do not have effective laboratory tests to measure most of these nutrients to see if a person has a deficiency. This section is really about the biochemistry of the cell. It gets complicated and the actual language that physiologists and biochemists use to discuss cellular activity requires a background to understand even the most basic of cellular function. I will discuss briefly the nutrients, fats, vitamins, minerals, phyto-nutrients, and amino acids involved in the cell physiology as well as herbs that secrete special growth factors which are important to healing the central nervous system.

Herbs:
This area of discussion is, as always problematic, as there are many varieties of each individual herb. For example, "Ginseng" has over eleven varieties. Should one use American, Korean, or Siberian ginseng? These are very important questions as each variety is different.

Each variety of ginseng has different ginsenosides (the active ingredient) and the content of these active ingredients depends on a number of factors, including the timing of the harvesting.

Remember, each company that provides herbal products, sell what they have, not what is necessarily the best product. This makes it very difficult for the consumer who wishes to purchase the best products.

Other effective herbs are panax ginseng, curcumin (an extract of turmeric), sylmarin, and milk thistle. These can be combined together as some are better for inflammation and some as anti-oxidants. The process is made simple for you by compounding the essential nutrients in NutraGen™ products.

Fats:
The low fat dietary recommendations given by the American Heart Association and the American Diabetes Association could well be the most devastating advice to patients the world over. As it turns out, every cell membrane in the body requires saturated fats to complete their membrane structure. These fats of course, are found in animal meats of all types. These saturated fats were

replaced with polyunsaturated vegetable oils, like soy oil, corn oil, safflower oil, etc. These oils are foreign to our systems and are pro-inflammatory, producing inflammatory chemokines which cause inflammation in the brain. They are products of modern food manufacturing designed for the convenience of the food industry only. They are not food stuffs that were ever available in the Paleolithic diet of our ancestors.

The cell membrane (over one trillion cells) in the body requires saturated fat to complete the structure and integrity of the membrane. They also require DHA/EPA (docosahexaenoic acid) essential fats that come from sea weed and fish oil, krill oil and certain natural sources like nuts. Forty percent of the fat in the brain is DHA.

The dry weight of the brain is about 50% fat. One can readily see that the proper types of fat are extremely important to supplement for proper neuron structure and function. In addition to flax, olive and coconut oil, other essential fats, and omega-3 fats in the proper ratio are also necessary for proper electrical conductivity of the cells in the brain. NutraGen™ has made a DHA/EPA product, Pure Omerga Plus™ that tastes good and contains the correct balance to give the brain the fat it needs to stay healthy.

Amino Acids:
Several proteins are necessray for the cell to function properly. Because proteins have an electrical charge, they are important in moving substances through the cell membrane and around the inside of the cell. In addition, the neurotransmitter substances that are responsible for communication between the cells are frequently proteins like dopamine, norepinephrine and serotonin, which are all derived from proteins. Carnitine, serene, glycine, threonine are necessary as they work inside of the cells, while

104

tryptophan and tyrosine are converted into neurotransmitters responsible for communication between the cells.

Neurotransmitters like GABA (gamma amino butyric acid), glutamate are also protein neurotransmitters. The major anti-oxidant in every cell is glutathione which is composed of three amino acids: glycine, cysteine and glutamic acid. N acetyl cysteine (NAC) is a very valuable amino acid not only because it is a necessary part of glutathione but because it contains a sulfur group. Hence it is active in liver detoxification and also in the nervous tissue where it performs multiple functions. So, one can see a wide variety of amino acids are required for proper brain function. Phosphatidylserine is a protein that enhances neurological function, and may have a profound influence in the patient with dementia. NutraGen™ Pure Cleanse Plus™ addresses these amino acids.

Only red meats contain all the essential amino acids for proper brain function. If you are a vegetarian, it is possible to get enough of essential proteins if you mix the various proteins like whey, pea, hemp and rice into your diet. NutraGen™ has developed a specialized protein supplement which can be made into a shake to supplement meat in your diet. This ensures you get enough protein in your diet to make the necessary neurotransmitters and to maintain muscle mass. Muscle maintenance is very important as seniors all suffer from sarcopenia, which is a loss of muscle mass. Remember I stated your muscles burn most of the calories you consume and if you have low muscle mass the calories cannot be burned and hence, you gain weight mostly as fat.

In addition, low muscle mass brings on frailty—the number one indicator of impending death. After the age of fifty, humans can lose 1-3% of their muscle mass per year, but these percentages are likely understated. Decreased neurotransmision from the brain to the muscles, age related hormonal loses, decreased protein intake, and lack of exercise are responsible for the muscle loss and accompanying frailty.

Minerals:
Minerals like copper, zinc, manganese, and iron are used in enzymes such as catalase and superoxide dismutase. Zinc and selenium deficiencies have recently found to be very important in neurological function. The cell combines these minerals with amino acids and hydrogen peroxide to manufacture enzymes which neutralize the damaging free radicals the result of cellular metabolism.

It is interesting to note that we still have not discovered exactly how enzymes like catalase and superoxide dismutase work—yet another mystery to be solved. Minerals like sodium, potassium, phosphorus, calcium, boron and magnesium all have an electrical charge and thus are active in transporting nutrients into and out of the brain cells.

Magnesium content inside of certain brain cells is dramatically altered and thus is associated with neuronal dysfunction. There seems to be an interference with aluminum in the neuronal cell (aluminum is toxic and not supposed to be in the brain) and this results in abnormal cellular metabolism. When aluminum combines with fluoride, it compounds the problem as it is very neuro toxic. Calcium is used by the astrocyte cells of the brain as a neurotransmitter substance enhancing communication between these specialized support cells of the brain. One can readily see that there is an important need to supplement these minerals, many of which are not readily available in our daily diet.

Vitamins:

Complex B vitamins because B complex vitamins, vitamin B^2 and B^3, are involved in every phase of the energy cycle of the cell, they are all vital to proper metabolism. B^{12} and folic acid are involved in a process called methylation. In this same process vitamin B^6 is a cofactor. These vitamins allow the cell to make the proteins necessary for DNA production, which allows the cell to control its internal messaging systems and to function properly. B^6 is required for all amino acid (protein) conversions.

Special forms of B Vitamins as I discussed in the drug section, some special forms are B^1 (benfotamine) and B^3 (niagen). These B complex vitamins are readily available in the NutraGen™ supplement and do not need to be converted by the body prior to usage by the body.

Choline as I have discussed is an essential nutrient in which most post-menopausal women are deficient. This nutrient is important as it is essential to the structure of the neuro-membrane, is a methyl donor and is an essential component of the neurotransmitter acetylcholine.

Inositol once thought to be in the B complex family, is very important to the membrane structure and to neurological conduction in the central nervous system.

CoQ10 is a vitamin like substance that is important to organelle function of every cell. It is involved in energy production of the cell and also acts as an antioxidant limiting oxidative stress.

Vitamin D was also discussed earlier and we are now well aware of its importance in brain function and its involvement in the immune response.

Vitamin E the most versatile fat soluble antioxidant is important not only inside of the cell, but within the membrane as well.

Vitamin C of course. The discussion would not be complete without mentioning Vitamin C. Some scientists have pointed out that humans cannot make their own vitamin C, and hence a shortage of C may well be why we cannot clear the amyloid plaques from our brains. Vitamin C may well be the most versatile anti-oxidant in the body and conservative estimates suggest we need much more than the suggested government recommended 60 milligrams daily. For good vitamin C balance, it is recommended to have an intake of three thousand milligrams daily taken throughout the day. It is water soluble and readily excreted through urine.

Phytonutrients:
Phytonutrients are small molecules that are derived from a number of natural sources. They often work as signal messengers that can affect entire systems or even multiple systems.

Resveratrol is a plant nutrient known for years to be found in red wine. It has been found to have a profound impact on blood glucose, so it has a positive effect on the liver function. In addition, it has a positive effect on the brain, perhaps assisting in the insulin resistance that occurs there. Research has proven it is an antioxidant affecting water soluble spaces in the cell and elsewhere.

Phytonutrients are sourced from plants, spices, beans, seeds, fruit, seaweed and herbs. They are often classified or referred to by their biochemical characteristics such as: polyphenols, procyanidins, genosenosides, catecthins, and polyphenolic acids. Some are active within the cell and some in the interstitial spaces between the cells. There are dozens of these that have been identified and have proven to be effective in human scientific studies as anti-inflammatory agents, anti-oxidants, blood purifiers, laxatives, glucose control agents, etc. Often times these compounds are more powerful than synthetic medications, but because they are derived from natural sources, patents by pharmaceutical companies are difficult to obtain. Phytonutrients likely work as the keys that are necessary to unlock the dysfunctional metabolism at the cellular level.

There are many of these polyphenols, genosenosides, catechins and other small plant molecules in the NutraGen™ Pure Greens™ product which act as signaling agents to assist the cell to reprogram its cellular function. This product is designed to provide optimal dosages of many of these compounds in order to provide support to the central nervous system.

—NOTES—

Stem Cells

In 2005, I began working with adult stem cells to treat patients for what I termed the "no option diseases." These diseases and conditions are those for which medicine does not have any effective medications or those where the patient has exhausted all treatment options.

Most of the chronic neurological diseases like Alzheimer's, Parkinson's disease, multiple sclerosis, and stroke, fall into the "no option diseases" category. Traumatic injuries to the brain (traumatic brain injury) and spine (spinal cord injury) are also included here as there is limited medical therapy for these problems.

Most patients get six months of physical therapy post injury and instruction on how to cope with their disability and that is all mainstream medicine has to offer.

After some success with Alzheimer's disease patients, using only stem cells, I have renewed hope that we can repair brain damage and rehabilitate patients towards a more functional state using stem cell therapy. We have in preclinical (animals models) significantly eliminated much of the plaque in genetic mice, (these are mice genetically programed to develop Alzheimer's).

After researching Alzheimer's, I found there were several possible causes for this disease and researchers were only addressing the sequelae (plaques and tangles) and not investigating what *caused* the plaques and tangles in the first place. I found much more was needed to address the etiology of the problem, since the causes are chronic and require long-term therapy.

Prior to the patient getting stem cells, I recommend a program to include the following:

- Cleaning up the underlying terrain of the body
- Detoxing the heavy metals
- Eliminating the spirochetes
- Cleansing the body of haloids-like fluoride
- Ensuring sufficient good nutrition, vitamins and anti-oxidants for the body to heal itself

This book has addressed these causal etiologies and briefly discussed an action plan that included several nutritional recommendations which must be implemented. This book informs the reader what the underlying causes are and how to eliminate exposure to them. The recommended supplements and diet give the body the essential nutrients to repair itself.

My program also addresses the inflammation in the brain which seems to be a universal problem in all neurological diseases. By utilizing anti-inflammatory nutrients and herbal formulas the viscous cycle of inflammation is broken. The mesenchymal stem cells also help to modulate the inflammation in the brain and have a dramatic effect on the inflammatory mediators after intravenous administration.

I firmly believe stem cell therapy is the foundation therapy for traumatic brain injury, diabetes, vascular dementia and Alzheimer's disease. These problems will have the best chance of responding to treatment as we set forth a comprehensive program of detox and instituting a neuro-regenerative program for healing.

Of course, recognizing that the best therapy is prevention and addressing the above conditions before full blown disease presents itself. By being proactive and starting the nutritional recommendations I have provided, even before there are symptoms of memory loss, will help prevent memory loss.

I have found while using stem cell therapy the doctor has to use the proper cells in order to achieve results. There is often a misconception even among doctors about which cells to use and one stem cell cannot do it all. I use nine different adult stem cell types in treating diseases

With Alzheimer's I use a neural stem cell, a mesenchymal stem cell and often times a muscle stem cell. Yes, three different types of adult stem cells. One type cannot address all the different systems that need healing.

Please see my book *Miracle of Stem Cells*. Of interest, as this book goes to press, there are 77 drug investigations under way to seek a treatment for Alzheimer's disease.

—NOTES—

PART FIVE

JumpStart

JumpStart Guide

When learning something new, it's not always easy to navigate on your own. A catalyst or helping hand to guide the way can be highly beneficial.

We have all jumpstarted a vehicle at one time or another where the battery is so dead the vehicle will not start on its own. Assistance is required. A forceful boost to help get going. The NutraGen™ JumpStart Guide is perfect for this initial and vigorous kick-off. And once set in motion you can proceed with more ease and confidence on your own.

The NutraGen™ JumpStart Guide has been designed to introduce lifestyle choices that are simple to make yet have a huge impact. The guide will direct you to make choices that facilitate the reduction of inflammation and stabilize your blood sugar— the two biggest instigators holding you back from achieving long lasting health.

Download 21 page JumpStart Guide for FREE from the NutraGen™ website www.nutragen.com. Refer to the site's home page tab "Free Programs".

The NutraGen™ Pure 28-Day Program of pre-formulated menus and balanced whole food selections, again FREE, will be found under the home page "Free Programs" as well. This 74 page download complements the JumpStart Guide.

—NOTES—

Getting Started

The following are some ideas on how to get started on your journey.

Finding a Doctor:
The first thing and by far the hardest, is to find a doctor. You, as a patient, do not have the time to educate them and if he or she is not interested in practicing "outside the box" which is what is needed in order to help you, <u>you will need to seek assistance and guidance elsewhere</u>. Unless your family doctor is an exceptional "out of the box" thinker, you will need an alternative medicine doctor. You can find one at:

- American College for Advancement of Medicine <u>www.acam.org</u>

- American Academy of Anti-aging Medicine, <u>www.A4M.com</u>

- Age Management Medicine Group, AMMG, <u>www.agemed.org</u>

If your state has Naturopathic doctors and Chiropractors who specialize in nutrition or clinical nutritionist that do nutritional consultations, they may also be able to help you.

Specialty Laboratories:
This lab information may be helpful to your doctor, they are not routine tests and specialize in new ways to look at diseased states.

- *Doctors Data*, www.doctorsdata.com is the lab I use to measure toxic metals levels, test stool samples for infectious agents in the gut, and allows us to measure good bacteria levels in the stool.

- *Genova Diagnostics*, www.gdx.net is the lab I use to measure hormones, including thyroid and vitamin D levels.

- *IGENEX Labs*, www.igenex.com is the standard to check for spirochetes (Lyme's disease). There is varying opinions as to which lab test is best, but this is the one that I use.

- *Singulex Labs*, www.singulex.com test for endothelial function. They have a panel of tests which allows the physician to evaluate endothelial function. Endothelin I, nitric oxide, and angiotensin II should also be measured, along with the traditional markers of homocysteine and hsCRP for endothelial health and inflammation.

Recommended Books on Diet:

There are several good books that I recommend that are basically a Paleo-type diet which eliminates all GMO foods, most starches with refined sugars and flour products. Fresh foods and red meats are recommended. The following are the diet books I recommend:

- *Blood Sugar Control* by Mark Hyman, MD

- *The Paleo Diet* by Loren Cordain, PhD

- *The Rosedale Diet* by Ron Rosedale, MD

- *Paleo Manifesto* by John Durant

- *The Big Fat Surprise* by Nina Teicholz

Remember, a diet low in refined carbohydrates (sugars and starches) and higher in *good* fats, proteins and complex carbohydrates is recommended.

For More Information:
If you have a loved one who is *showing signs* or *you* are worried that you may be suffering from forgetfulness and looming dementia, NutraGen™ has compiled a list of nutritional supplements. These supplements are designed to make it simple to assist you in your fight against Alzheimer's disease. See JumpStart formulas at www.nutragen.com.

Medical research tells us that if you have had a stroke, traumatic brain injury or Parkinson's disease, you are very likely to experience dementia in the course of your life. Now is the time to initiate a plan of action which will either delay, or even prevent the onset of dementia.

To learn more about stem cell treatment, you can visit my web site at www.stemcells4life.net. To get a list of nutritionals specifically targeted to assist the body in its recovery from Alzheimer's. You may contact me at info@stemcells4life.net.

— NOTES —

Check List

1) Find a doctor – see list of doctor organizations to find a doctor that thinks "outside of the box".

2) Do the memory tests on the website: www.alzheimersreadingroom.com/p/test-your-memory-for - alzheimers-5-best.html.

3) Labs and other tests that you will need:

   - Comprehensive stool assessment

   - Complete hormone panel

   - Blood test for spirochetes

   - Oral spirochete and bacterial test

   - Heavy metals test edta/dmps challenge test

   - Vascular and systemic markers of inflammation, include ApoE4 test

   - Thyroid exam full panel including rT3 (reverse T3) test

   - Routine blood work including blood lipids, liver panel, HbA1C, electrolytes

4) Doctor appointment. This appointment is very important. Before you even start an exam, show the doctor a list of the tests and outline your goals (best to purchase this book for him) and ask, will he:

- Order the tests

- Help you balance your hormones

- Treat any toxicity found on the labs

- Rebalance your colon flora

- Help you to treat blood sugar problems, diabetes and endothelial dysfunction

- Give you a mental status exam for a base line

5) Find a biological knowledgeable dentist.

- Develop a plan to get all of the metals out of your mouth this includes amalgam fillings, posts, and root canal teeth, removed. Have the dentist do any filling with bio compatible materials.

- Get a laser treatment on the teeth and gums to kill the biofilms.

- Dentures may be necessary if too much work is needed.

- Get your mouth tested for spirochetes and other bacteria.

6) There are several organizations that may help you find the right dentist. Refer to Appendix, Resources for websites.

- *International Academy of Biological Dentistry* educates dentists, physicians, and other practitioners.

- *Holistic Dental Association* which offers support to both consumers and holistic dentists.

- *International Academy of Oral Medicine and Toxicology* which has taken the lead in educating dentists in safely dealing with amalgam fillings, and in developing more biocompatible approaches in other areas of dentistry, including endodontics, periodontics, and disease prevention. You'll be looking for a member in your area.

- Dr. Tom McGuire also keeps a *Directory of Dentists* who do not use mercury in their fillings.

—NOTES—

Products

Your ability to perform physically and mentally depends on getting enough quality nutrients in the right balance.

Inflammation is the hallmark of neuro-degenerative diseases. NutraGen™ products contain therapeutic doses designed to reduce inflammation and provide the high quality nutrients necessary to achieve proper balance. The NutraGen™ Solution to Chronic Inflammation can be found at www.nutragen.com.

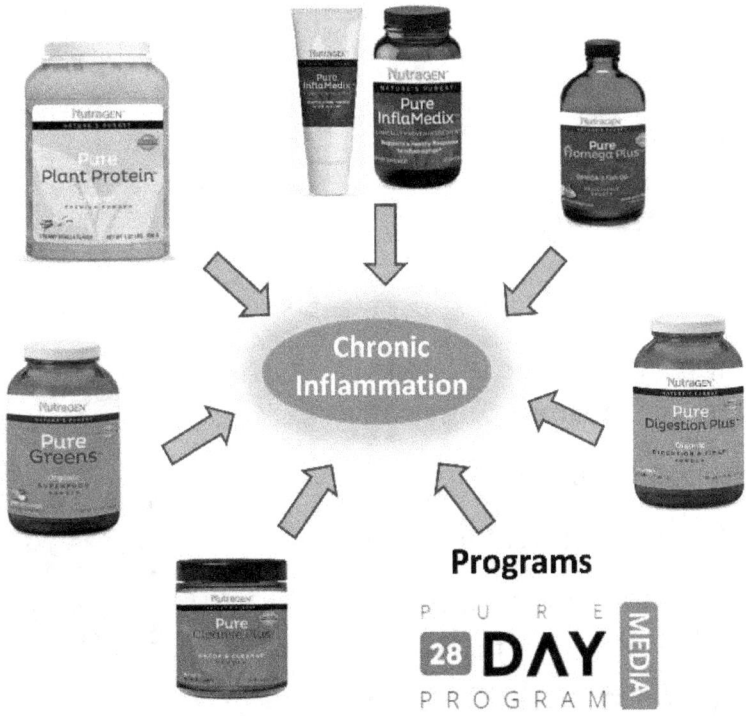

Daily Lifestyle Inflammation Program:
I recommend you take each of the following products on a daily basis, along with the Daily Inflammation Kit. This program is designed for those that desire maximum natural solution to reducing inflammation and achieving a healthy lifestyle:

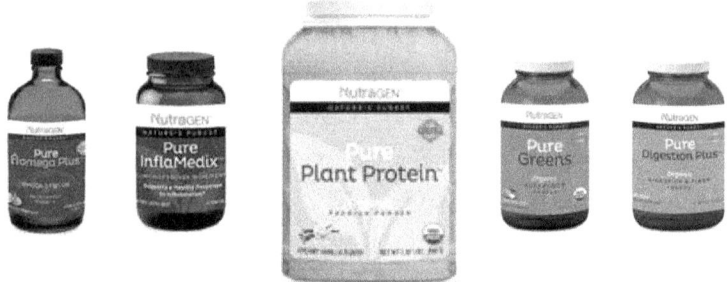

Pure InflaMedix™:
Unregulated inflammation may be at the root of most common chronic diseases of aging, including cancer, heart disease, Alzheimer's, diabetes and arthritis. Extensive clinical research on the ingredients in Pure InflaMedix™ has been shown to regulate the normal inflammatory process by targeting and inhibiting the pro-inflammatory enzymes.

Pure InflaMedix™ contains therapeutic doses to support:

- Healthy response to acute and chronic inflammation

- Cognitive function and memory

- Healthy joints and flexibility

- Temporary relief for muscle aches and soreness from active lifestyles

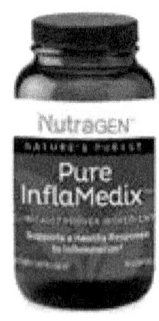

Pure Aomega Plus™:
Do you eat enough fish, nuts, flax, and leafy greens on a daily basis for optimal health? Pure Aomega Plus™ comes in a delicious, creamy citrus-mango flavor and does NOT smell, taste, or repeat like other fish oils. It also provides organic turmeric, vitamin D3, and astaxanthin for additional inflammation, antioxidant, and bone support.

Pure Aomega Plus™ contains therapeutic doses to support:

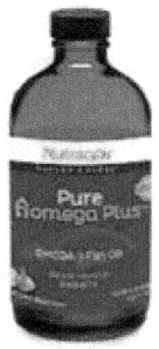

- Response to inflammation

- Brain

- Bone & joints

- Skin & hair

Daily Inflammation Kit:
These products are designed to be taken on a daily basis. The daily recommended dose for the Inflammation Kit is two capsules per day with food of the Pure InflaMedix™ and one tablespoon per day of Pure Aomega Plus™.

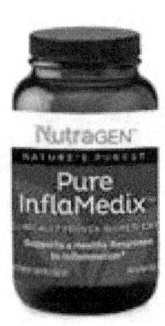 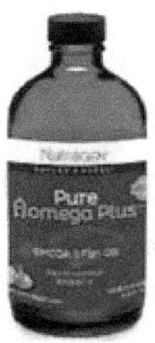

Crisis Care:

In the event you are in extreme pain or suffering from severe inflammation, I would categorize you as crisis care. I would recommend you see your Health Practitioner and the following treatment program:

Pure InflaMedix™
Week 1: 3 capsules 3 x per day with food
Week 2: 3 capsules 3 x per day with food
Week 3: 2 capsules 2 x per day with food
Thereafter: 2 capsules per day (ongoing for maintenance)

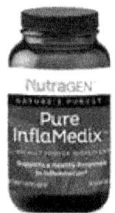

Pure Aomega Plus™
Week 1:   1 tablespoon 3 x per day
Week 2-3: 1 tablespoon 2 x per day
Thereafter: 1 tablespoon per day
(ongoing for maintenance)

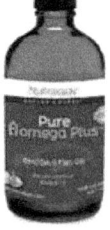

Proteins:

Pure Plant Protein™ is easily digested and perfectly balanced with the cleanest, highest quality organic protein blend. It blends well with the other NutraGen™ products to create a delicious, nutrient dense, low calorie meal replacement shake.

Pure Plant Protein™ contains therapeutic doses to support:

- Energy, strength & focus

- Weight loss/weight management

- Muscle repair & maintenance

- Blood sugar stability

- Healthy response to inflammation

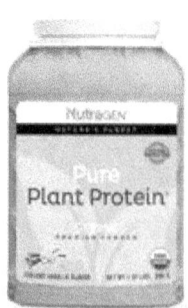

Fruits and Vegetables:

Do you eat the recommended 7 to 10 servings of fruits, vegetables and leafy greens each day? If not, take the next best thing... Pure Greens™ has been expertly crafted with organic, gluten-free grass juices, vegetables, fruits, herbs and plants to assist you in meeting your daily requirements.

Pure Greens™ contains therapeutic doses to support:

- Blood sugar stability

- Immune system

- Enhanced alkalinity

- Increased antioxidant levels

- Cognitive function and memory

- Healthy response to inflammation

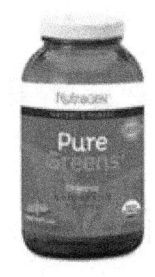
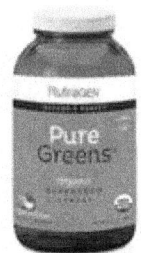

Fiber and Digestion:

Do you eat the recommended 25-35 grams of fiber each day? Fiber deficiency is associated with poor digestion, fatigue, obesity, diabetes and heart disease. Pure Digestion Plus™ delivers 12 grams of organic fibers in each serving and blends well in water or in a shake. It also provides probiotics, digestive enzymes, papaya, and perilla leaf for enhanced digestive support.

Pure Digestion Plus™ contains therapeutic doses to support:

- Healthy digestion & regularity

- Reduction of abdominal discomfort, including pain, cramps & bloating

- Blood sugar stability

- Healthy response to inflammation

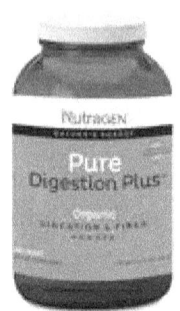

Detoxification:

Pure Cleanse Plus™ has been designed to assist your body in clearing metabolic waste and environmental toxins such as heavy metals, pesticides, herbicides, solvents and drug residues. If you are suffering from acne, rosacea, brain fog, stress, fatigue, depression, weight loss resistance, acid reflux, irritable bowel, achy muscles and joints, blood sugar instability or diabetes, Pure Cleanse Plus™ may benefit you.

Pure Cleanse Plus™ is a new comprehensive detoxification formula that contains therapeutic doses to support:

- Complete liver and organ detoxification

- Elimination of environmental and metabolic toxins

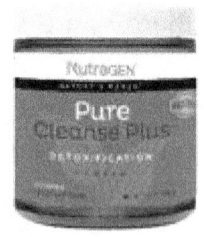

- Healthy response to inflammation

- Normal blood glucose levels

- Weight loss and lean muscle mass

Maximum Detoxification Program (28 Day Program):
I recommend everyone to complete a full detoxification one to two times per year. The program includes each of our products (some taken twice per day and some once per day), healthy eating, exercise, and sleep. This 28 Day Program is designed for individuals that require:

- Complete liver and organ detoxification
- Elimination of environmental and metabolic toxins

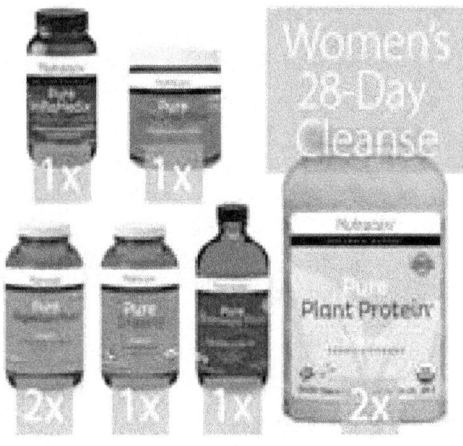

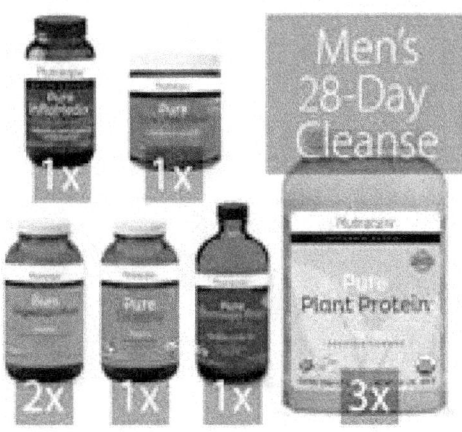

—NOTES—

APPENDIX

Glossary

Amyloid—incorrectly folded protein fibre (elongated threadlike nerve cells). When an amyloid protein folds abnormally, an insoluble fibre called a fibril is formed. If several fibrils clump together they create plaque in the brain.

Antigen—a toxin or other foreign substance causing an immune response in the body.

Apolipoprotein—proteins that transport lipids (fat and cholesterol) through the lymphatic and circulatory systems of the body.

Casual Association—noxious peripheral agent that has some influence or role in producing the occurrence of a disease.

Cribriform plate—bone at the notch of the frontal bone and roofs in the nasal cavities.

Endothelial tissue—the inside lining of blood vessels.

Etiology—study of why things occur along with the reasons behind the way things act.

Genome—full DNA sequence of an organism or more specifically the human body.

Haloid—resembling a salt and readily form negative ions to become toxic as a radical element attaching to healthy ions causing body deterioration.

Hapten—small molecule that can elicit an immune response from the body when attached to a large carrier such as a protein.

In vivo—in a living organism. For example, an experiment that is done in vivo is done in the body of a living organism as opposed to in a laboratory method that does not use the living organism as the host of the test. In vivo is the opposite of in vitro.

Macrophages—scavengers, they rid the body of worn-out cells and other debris. They play a crucial role in initiating an immune response.

Magnetic resonance imaging (MRI)—test using a machine to pulse radio wave energy throughout the body to make pictures of organs and structures inside the body.

Medical Models—set of procedures in which all doctors are trained for their medical research.

Mentation—process of using your mind to consider something carefully.

Metabolic syndrome—collection of symptoms that can lead to diabetes and heart disease. Such symptoms include high blood pressure, obesity, high cholesterol, and insulin resistance.

Microglia—type of cell that act as the first and main form of active immune defense in the central nervous system

Myelin—insulating material that forms a layer, the myelin sheath, usually around only the axon of a neuron and essential for the proper functioning of the nervous system.

Neurogenesis—process by which neurons are generated from neural stem cells.

Oligodendrocytes— main function is to provide support and insulation to axons in the central nervous system.

Phthalates—substances added to plastics to increase their flexibility, transparency, durability, and longevity.

Phytonutrients—nutrients derived from plant material shown to be necessary for sustaining human life.

Reserve Capacity—ability of the brain to optimize or maximize its performance by using alternative brain networks to maintain cognitive functions.

Sequelae—condition encountered from the consequences of a previous disease or injury.

Spirochetes—type of bacteria that does not have a nucleus, most have corkscrew-shaped cells hence the name.

Vascular dementia—dementia caused by problems in the supply of blood to the brain, typically by a series of minor strokes.

—NOTES—

Sources for Further Research

The following sources were referred to often in the writing of this book and have been mentioned throughout the book. They are highlighted again in one place for ease of reference. I highly encourage my readers to further their quest to enrich their life by doing extended research and investigation. This list is only a start.

Diet:

The Blood Sugar Solution 10-Day Detox Diet Cookbook by Mark Hyman, MD. More than 150 Recipes to Help You Lose Weight and Stay Healthy for Life. Published 2015.

Ketogenic Diet 101 www.authoritynutrition.com/ketogenic-diet-101 article by Rudy Mawer, MSc, CISSN "A Detailed Beginner's Guide" listing foods to avoid and foods to eat. A real wealth of information on healthy eating in general.

The Paleo Diet by Loren Cordain, PhD. Lose Weight and Get Healthy by Eating the Foods You Were Designed to Eat. Published 2010.

The Paleo Manifesto: Ancient Wisdom for Lifelong Health by John Durant. From diet to movement to sleep, this evolutionary perspective sheds light on some of our most pressing health concerns. Published 2014.

The Rosedale Diet: Turn Off Your Hunger Switch by Ron Rosedale, MD. Based on more than twenty years of research and the latest findings on appetite and weight. Published 2006.

Directories:

International Academy of Biological Dentistry www.iabdm.org website dedicated to educating dentists, physicians, and other practitioners with a referral directory.

Holistic Dental Association www.holisticdental.org providing support and guidance to practitioners of holistic and alternative dentistry since 1978. Offers support to both consumers and holistic dentists. Has listing of Holistic Dentists.

International Academy of Oral Medicine and Toxicology www.iaomt.org promotes biological dental medicine utilizing non-toxic diagnostic and therapeutic approaches in the field of clinical dentistry. Education in dealing with amalgam fillings. Member physician listing.

Directory of Dentists www.dentalwellness4u.com Dr. Tom McGuire's mercury safe dentists' internet directory.

Environment:

Environmental Working Group EWG.org motto "know your environment, protect your health" keeps its readers up to date on the latest findings in environmental health issues. A site worth bookmarking and sourcing on a continual basis.

Labs and Diagnostics:

Cyrex Laboratories www.joincyrex.com tests designed to detect and monitor autoimmune reactivity's and their possible triggers specifically for food allergies and other environmental triggers along with barrier permeability (intestinal and brain) and identification of markers and possible precursors to autoimmune disorder.

Doctors Data www.doctorsdata.com test designed to measure toxic metals levels, and test stool samples for infectious agents in the gut and good bacteria levels in the stool.

Genova Diagnostics www.gdx.net tests designed to provide a more complete understanding of specific biological systems that can help physicians diagnose and treat or prevent chronic disease.

IGENEX Labs www.igenex.com test designed to ascertain the presence of Lyme disease.

Immunosciences Lab, Inc. www.immunoscienceslab.com menu of tests used to support diagnostics of autoimmune diseases. Contact for a catalog of services and testing panels.

Singulex Labs www.singulex.com blood tests designed to give early detection of possible disease and indication of health.

SpectraCell Laboratories www.SpectraCell.com nutritional and cardiometabolic testing assessing a spectrum of risk factors and biomarkers for optimum wellness.

ZRT Laboratory www.zrtlab.com hormone testing available in a selection of specialty profiles. Each profile is geared to specific health conditions.

Products:

NutraGen™ www.nutragen.com as mentioned throughout my book, doctor designed supplements: Pure Plant Protein™, Pure Greens™, Pure Digestion Plus™ and Pure Aomega Plus™. The JumpStart Guide and the Pure 28-Day Program are both free and can be found under "Free Programs" website home page tabs.

Pulsed Electrical Magnetic Frequency (PEMF)
www.DrPawluk.com healing with magnetic field energy is recommended for all neurological conditions as they reconnect your body with the frequencies of the earth.

Stemedica Cell Technology www.stemedica.com a biopharmaceutical company that develops and manufactures adult stem cell products for use in clinical and pre-clinical trials.

Self-Testing and Development:

Alzheimer's Test ww.alzheimersreadingroom.com/p/test-your-memory-for-alzheimers-5-best.html download test to take on your own.

Brain+ www.brain-plus.com digital therapeutics for cognitive remediation with downloadable apps to exercise and engage your brain via therapist support or as self-care.

About the Author
David A. Howe, MD, DC

Dr. David A. Howe brings over 35 years of executive leadership experience as a medical director and clinical doctor. He championed the design, development and implementation of solutions related to the advancement of stem cell technology while contributing significantly to all critical processes and procedures from the laboratory to clinical practice.

Dr. Howe serves as a "subject matter" expert to various regulatory and medical agencies in over twelve countries, each involved in various stages of stem cell treatment and research. He provides advisory services to government, regulatory, hospital medical and technical teams, ethics and Investigational Review Boards. Co-author of the authoritative book on stem cells entitled *The Miracle of Stem Cells: How Adult Stem Cells Are Transforming Lives,* Dr. Howe is available for presentations.

As the Chief Executive and Medical Officer at "Longevity Medicine" center, Dr. Howe incorporates innovations in science and technology designed to significantly improve quality of life, increase life expectancy and to enhance the well-being of people of all ages. To achieve these objectives, the Longevity Medicine Center brings together the best minds in longevity and regenerative medicine, stem cell research and therapy, nutritional consultation, and physical and rehabilitative therapies.

Dr. Howe is one of the co-founders of Stemedica Cell Technologies, Inc., a world leading bio-pharmaceutical company specializing in developing, manufacturing and distributing multiple lines of allogeneic adult stem cell products (for human use) that are used to treat a variety of diseases and medical conditions. Between 2005 and 2011, he served as Senior Vice President and Medical Director.

Dr. Howe provided oversight as a senior strategist, innovator and implementer in championing the design, development and implementation of ethical guidelines and clinical protocols for stem cell technologies used for treatment and for regulatory agency approval. He has collaborated with world renowned stem cell scientists, physicians and technicians in developing quality systems, protocols and best practices in stem cell translational medicine.

Dr. Howe advocates for, and provides strategic and tactical direction, in the adoption of innovative systems and processes to support infrastructure, medical informatics concepts, expertise, and knowledge required for integration with clinical and business needs. He has co-led the clinical studies, analysis of data and report generation related to various medical diseases and conditions. He has participated in the preparation of outcome data used in the application for regulatory approvals in over twelve countries.

Prior to his role at Stemedica, Dr. Howe was the owner and Medical Director of the San Diego Clinic of Preventive Medicine, which specializes in the most current treatments using alternative as well as mainstream medicine.

Dr. Howe received his Medical Degree from Ross University in New York City, and his Doctor of Chiropractic from the National

146

College of Chiropractic Medicine in Chicago, Illinois. Dr. Howe received a Master's Degree in Business Administration from St. Thomas University in St. Paul, Minnesota.

Since 2005, Dr. Howe has participated in advanced, post-doctoral training specializing in the science, development, manufacturing, protocol development and transplantation of adult stem cells at the Presidents Kremlin Hospital, the Federov Eye Institute & the Institute of General Pathology and Pathophysiology in Moscow, Russia.

Dr. Howe has personally been involved in the stem cell treatment of over 300 patients from the United States and abroad with medical diseases and conditions related to neurology, ophthalmology, cardiology and dermatology. Dr. Howe has personally participated in stem cell studies and has been a recipient of stem cell transplantation.